Chronic
Heartburn

Chronic Heartburn

Managing Acid Reflux and GERD Through Understanding, Diet and Lifestyle

Barbara E. Wendland, MSc, RD,
and Lisa Marie Ruffolo

> To Olga, Rose and Elizabeth
> —Barbara E. Wendland
>
> To anyone who has ever experienced the pain of heartburn
> —Lisa Marie Ruffolo

The authors would like to thank the following for sharing their knowledge and expertise during the writing of this book: David Armstrong, MD, FRCPC, Gastroenterology, McMaster University; Barry H. Shrott, MD.

This book is a general guide only and should never be a substitute for the skill, knowledge, and experience of a qualified medical professional dealing with the facts, circumstances, and symptoms of a particular case.

The nutritional, medical, and health information presented in this book is based on the research, training, and professional experience of the authors, and is true and complete to the best of their knowledge. However, this book is intended only as an informative guide for those wishing to know more about health, nutrition, and medicine; it is not intended to replace or countermand the advice given by the reader's personal physician. Because each person and situation is unique, the authors and the publisher urge the reader to check with a qualified health-care professional before using any procedure where there is a question as to its appropriateness. A physician should be consulted before beginning any exercise program. The authors and the publisher are not responsible for any adverse effects or consequences resulting from the use of the information in this book. It is the responsibility of the reader to consult a physician or other qualified health-care professional regarding his or her personal care.

Editors: Bob Hilderley, Senior Editor, Health; and Sue Sumeraj
Recipe tester: Jennifer MacKenzie
Copy editor and proofreader: Sheila Wawanash
Index: Gillian Watts
Design and production: PageWave Graphics Inc.
Cover photography: Mark T. Shapiro
Illustration: Kveta / Three in a Box

The publisher acknowledges the financial support of the Government of Canada through the Book Publishing Industry Development Program (BPIDP).

Published by Robert Rose Inc.
120 Eglinton Ave. E., Suite 800, Toronto, Ontario Canada M4P 1E2
Tel: (416) 322-6552 Fax: (416) 322-6936

Printed and bound in Canada

1 2 3 4 5 6 7 8 9 CPL 14 13 12 11 10 09 08 07 06

Contents

Preface

Heartburn as a result of acid reflux can be incredibly frustrating and persistently painful. For some people, heartburn is merely the symptom of a minor intermittent problem, but for others, it is the symptom of a major chronic condition known as gastrointestinal reflux disease. The purpose of our book is to provide a source of information on this condition, explaining why you experience chronic heartburn, when you should seek medical treatment, and how to incorporate lifestyle changes, especially changes to your diet, so you can manage painful and annoying symptoms.

If you have symptoms of chronic heartburn, this book will help you learn more about the disorder and gain relief from the pain you are experiencing. Questions to be answered include the following:

- What are the symptoms, causes, and complications of chronic heartburn?
- Who is vulnerable to the development of acid reflux problems?
- When do you need to involve your doctor?
- What role does medication play in managing acid reflux?
- What lifestyle changes can be made to relieve chronic heartburn?
- What is the best diet to provide relief and prevent chronic heartburn?
- What recipes are best for chronic heartburn?

Start by reading the first chapters on the symptoms and causes of heartburn. If you are eager to understand more about medical therapies for treating chronic heartburn, move on to those chapters. At any time go to the diet and recipe sections. Foods that potentially aggravate or relieve symptoms are identified. Sample menus are presented based on the severity of symptoms. And more than 100 recipes are included that we have created and tested for managing acid reflux. These recipes are well tolerated if you are sensitive to acid and other irritating ingredients. Meals can be a comfortable and enjoyable experience — even when you have chronic heartburn. Use the recipes to take control of your symptoms as you regain your optimum health.

Healing Chronic Heartburn

Heartburn Basics

CHAPTER 1

What Is Heartburn?

Case History: Dan

Dan is a 47-year-old owner of a hardware store who has awakened at 2:00 a.m. with a burning feeling in his chest area, just behind the breastbone, and a sour taste in the back of his throat. This has been happening periodically for quite a few months now, and he has been taking antacid tablets before going to bed to help with this heartburn. While the antacid tablets provide some relief, they are no longer acting as rapidly or for as long. When he sits up, he feels some relief, but for the rest of the night Dan gets little rest. He continually feels the need to clear his throat.

The pain has become exhausting; the lack of restful sleep makes each day something of an ordeal. Dan's quality of life has been gradually decreasing over the past year as a result of this ongoing problem, and the situation is getting worse. His symptoms used to occur mainly after meals and at night, but now he begins experiencing pain most of the time, with changes in severity throughout the day. He also feels pain in his back. Sometimes, the pain is so severe that Dan fears he is having a heart attack.

When he finally visits his doctor, Dan is diagnosed with chronic heartburn or, as his doctor says, "gastroesophageal reflux disease," sometimes abbreviated as GERD.

(continued, page 22)

Heartburn is a common symptom of gastroesophageal reflux (GER), a digestive disorder that is the result of an abnormal backflow of acidic juices from the stomach up into the esophagus. In addition to a burning sensation felt in the chest, this acid reflux is experienced as a sour taste in the throat area and sometimes as chest pain. Many sufferers also experience regurgitation — a feeling that stomach contents have risen into the back of the throat or mouth. These symptoms of acid reflux are not only relatively common among the general population but also increasingly common during the past two decades, especially in Western nations, for reasons that are not yet clear.

If these symptoms persist and become chronic, the result may be a disease condition called gastroesophageal reflux disease (GERD). While not life-threatening, these symptoms seriously affect quality of life and may require, in the worst-case scenario, surgical intervention. There are many possible treatments for this condition, including popular over-the-counter and prescription drugs, but people with severe symptoms do not always respond favorably. Increasingly, health-care professionals are looking to diet as both a possible cause and an effective treatment for chronic heartburn.

Working Terms

Heartburn: The common term given to a symptom of a gastroesophageal reflux, where stomach "acids" back up into the esophagus and cause a burning sensation in the chest. Although most people experience heartburn occasionally, the symptom becomes chronic when experienced several times a week on a regular basis.

Acid Reflux: An abbreviated term for gastroesophageal reflux, with "acid" referring to the digestive juices that back up from the stomach to the esophagus.

Gastroesophageal Reflux (GER): The medical term used to describe the symptoms of heartburn and acid reflux that might occur from time to time to anyone, perhaps after a heavy meal, when food might be moving very slowly out of the stomach.

Gastroesophageal Reflux Disease (GERD): When these symptoms continue to occur on a regular basis, with a frequency of more than twice a week, and interfere with quality of life, the term "disease" is added to describe this chronic condition.

Heartburn Origins

Heartburn is a digestive disorder that occurs when the normal process of digestion goes wrong.

Did You Know...

Heartburn is not a rare symptom and acid reflux is a common disorder. Data from the United States suggest that about 44% of the population experiences acid reflux at least once a month, while about 20% of the population experiences related symptoms at least once a week. Recent data from a Canadian survey suggest that about 17% of the population experiences heartburn from time to time, while about 13% indicated that they experienced significant, often severe, heartburn at least once a week.

The primary role of the digestive tract is to process food, enabling the body to benefit from nutrients and fluids that are essential for survival. Under normal circumstances, the movement of food throughout the digestive tract occurs without our conscious awareness. We consume food, it moves through the digestive system, and we eliminate the waste materials. Normally, the digestive tract proceeds with its usual functions without our awareness.

However, sometimes we become aware of how our digestive tract is functioning if the passage of food causes a gurgling noise, if indigestion causes stomach upset, or if bloating occurs, perhaps due to excessive intake or stomach gas. We also become aware of our digestive system when we experience heartburn and other symptoms of gastroesophageal reflux.

Digestive Process

The actual movement of food through the digestive system occurs as a result of signals to nerves and muscles that work together in an organized and regulated manner to enable the movement of food through the digestive tract.

Mouth

The digestion of food begins within the mouth, where enzymes begin to break down some of the food. Saliva in the mouth helps the food to stick together, facilitating movement from the throat down toward the stomach. Usually, food and liquids move from the mouth, through the esophagus and into the stomach in an orderly manner, assisted by the effect of gravity and pushed by the wavelike muscular action of the esophagus, called peristalsis.

Esophagus

The act of swallowing has a direct effect on relaxing and opening valve-like muscles or sphincters in the esophagus. As food is being swallowed, a tight valve-like muscle at the top of the esophagus relaxes, enabling passage into the esophagus. This upper esophageal sphincter (UES) muscle then closes. Within the esophagus, smooth muscle contractions, called peristaltic waves, guide food toward the stomach.

At the junction of the esophagus and the stomach there is another valvelike muscle, called the lower esophageal

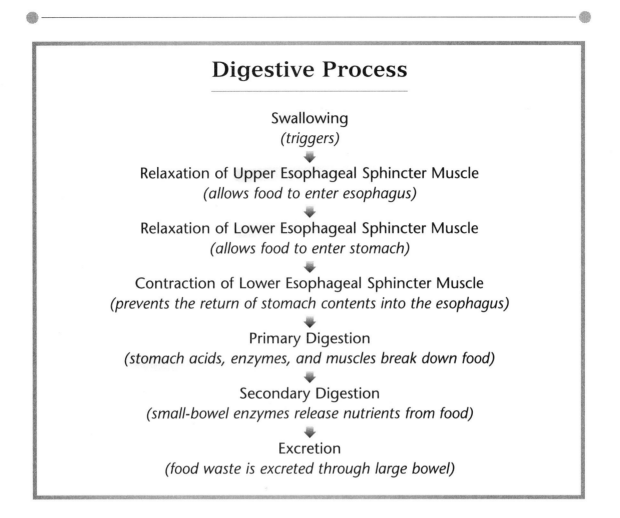

Digestive Process

Swallowing
(triggers)

Relaxation of Upper Esophageal Sphincter Muscle
(allows food to enter esophagus)

Relaxation of Lower Esophageal Sphincter Muscle
(allows food to enter stomach)

Contraction of Lower Esophageal Sphincter Muscle
(prevents the return of stomach contents into the esophagus)

Primary Digestion
(stomach acids, enzymes, and muscles break down food)

Secondary Digestion
(small-bowel enzymes release nutrients from food)

Excretion
(food waste is excreted through large bowel)

sphincter (LES), that is tightly controlled. To enable the passage of food into the stomach, the lower esophageal sphincter begins to relax. This muscle then contracts and closes to prevent a reflux, or backup, of acidic digestive juices from the stomach into the esophagus. This valve also allows excess gas to escape by belching or burping, lowering pressure in the stomach.

Stomach

The stomach acts like a reservoir where the primary digestive activity begins on food. The stomach produces digestive juices, chiefly hydrochloric acid and pepsin enzymes, to break down and sterilize the food we eat. With the assistance of the muscular action of the stomach, these digestive juices transform food from a solid form into a semi-liquid texture. When the digestive system is working normally, these acidic digestive juices remain in the stomach.

Digestive System

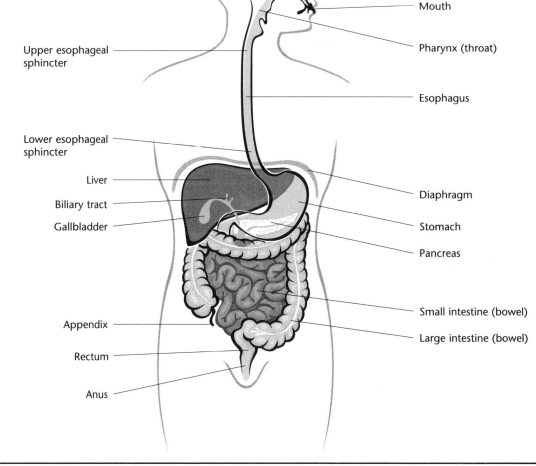

Mouth

Pharynx (throat)

Upper esophageal sphincter

Esophagus

Lower esophageal sphincter

Liver

Biliary tract

Gallbladder

Diaphragm

Stomach

Pancreas

Small intestine (bowel)

Appendix

Large intestine (bowel)

Rectum

Anus

Bowels

Once the digested food has reached the desired consistency, it is then moved out of the stomach via another valve-like muscle, the pyloric sphincter, into the small bowel. Within the small bowel, additional digestive enzymes work on the food. Eventually, nutrients released from the digestive action on food are absorbed within the small bowel and food waste is eliminated through the large bowel.

Reflux

Most people do experience some degree of acid reflux on occasion, despite the tightly regulated system of moving food into the stomach and then closing off the lower esophageal sphincter. The body has a means to correct this. Normally, the reflux of acid from the stomach into the esophagus will stimulate muscle contractions within the esophagus to push acid back into the stomach. Swallowed saliva and bicarbonate, secreted by the esophagus, are both alkaline and can neutralize the effect of refluxed acid in the esophagus.

If the lower esophageal sphincter muscle is working normally, it should prevent reflux and protect the esophagus from damage caused by acid pepsin and bile. Reflux only becomes a problem when there are clear and troublesome symptoms, such as frequent excessive amounts of acid refluxed into the esophagus that are not forced back into the stomach. This reflux of acidic digestive juices into the esophagus is what causes the burning pain and the sour acid taste in the throat.

Failure of this physiological anti-reflux mechanism gives rise to the symptoms of gastroesophageal reflux, including heartburn, and injury to the esophagus characteristic of gastroesophageal reflux disease. The lower esophageal sphincter that controls the passage of food between the lower esophagus and the stomach loses its tone and is unable to prevent the backflow of acidic digestive juices.

When the lower esophageal sphincter valve does not work as expected, other things can start to happen as a result of the open LES valve:

- Acid and digestive juices from the stomach back up into the esophagus through the open valve, often causing severe irritation to the delicate tissue of the esophagus.
- Chronic irritation to the esophageal tissue can lead to the severe inflammation and wearing away of the tissue, which might result in painful ulcers.
- Sometimes the inflamed tissue of the esophagus becomes so irritated that bleeding occurs.
- Chronic tissue irritation can lead to scar tissue formation, which causes narrowing of the esophagus, making the passage of food more difficult.
- Sometimes the chronic inflammation and ongoing irritation of tissue result in changes in the actual esophageal tissue to a pre-cancerous state that may eventually lead to esophageal cancer.

Did You Know...

Most people experience acid reflux from time to time. Acid reflux only becomes a problem when there are clear and troublesome symptoms that occur with it.

How the Esophagus Works

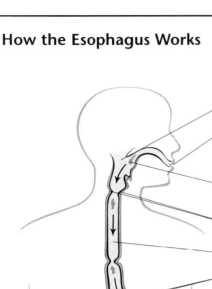

- Pharynx (throat)
- Mouth
- Food
- Upper esophageal sphincter
- Esophagus
- Lower esophageal sphincter
- Diaphragm
- Stomach

As food is being swallowed, it moves from the mouth into the throat, or pharynx. A tight valve-like muscle, or sphincter, at the top of the esophagus relaxes, enabling passage into the esophagus. The upper esophageal sphincter muscle then closes, and within the esophagus, smooth muscle contractions, called peristaltic waves, guide food toward the stomach. At the junction of the esophagus and the stomach, there is another valve-like muscle that is tightly controlled, the lower-esophageal sphincter (LES). This muscle closely regulates the entry of food into the stomach.

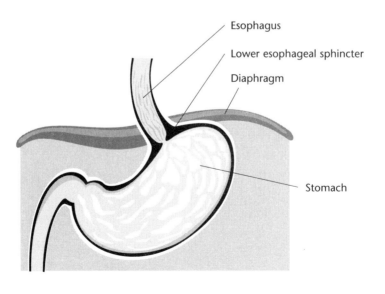

- Esophagus
- Lower esophageal sphincter
- Diaphragm
- Stomach

How Reflux Works

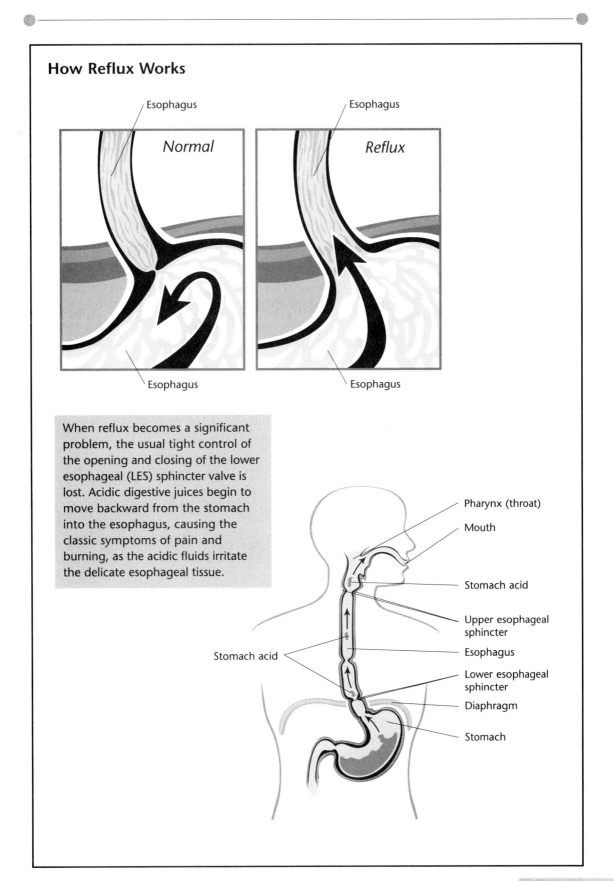

Esophagus

Normal

Esophagus

Esophagus

Reflux

Esophagus

When reflux becomes a significant problem, the usual tight control of the opening and closing of the lower esophageal (LES) sphincter valve is lost. Acidic digestive juices begin to move backward from the stomach into the esophagus, causing the classic symptoms of pain and burning, as the acidic fluids irritate the delicate esophageal tissue.

Pharynx (throat)

Mouth

Stomach acid

Upper esophageal sphincter

Stomach acid

Esophagus

Lower esophageal sphincter

Diaphragm

Stomach

Symptoms of Gastroesophageal Reflux

- Heartburn (a burning sensation behind the breast bone)
- Regurgitation (a feeling of food or liquids rising to the back of the throat or mouth)
- Taste of acid in the back of the throat
- Feeling of severe chest pain (not related to the heart)
- Pain not only in the chest area, but also in the back
- Upper abdominal pain with a burning feeling and nausea
- Problem with swallowing that accompanies the heartburn and acid reflux
- Chronic cough with a need to keep clearing the throat
- Hoarseness of the voice or laryngitis

Q: How do I know if I have gastroesophageal reflux disease?

A: Have you experienced the key problems of heartburn and a sour taste of acid in the back of your throat on a regular basis?

Have you taken over-the-counter medications, such as Tums, Zantac, or Pepcid, on a regular basis to help control your symptoms?

If the answer is "Yes" to both of these questions, you may have a problem with this disease.

Did You Know...

Some people develop pre-cancerous tissue changes in the area around the LES, a condition called Barrett's esophagus. This condition needs to be monitored closely for potential development of cancer.

Health Complications

Up to 40% to 50% of the population has heartburn at least once a month that readily responds to over-the-counter medication and lifestyle modifications, such as discontinuing cigarette use, reducing alcohol consumption, and working at increasing overall health using diet, physical activity, and stress management. These measures may alleviate heartburn and other symptoms of gastroesophageal reflux. However, sometimes these symptoms can become more severe and lead to serious health complications.

Chronic Inflammation

In the long term, some people develop persistent problems with acid reflux that can result in the development of a more severe chronic inflammatory reaction. Acidic digestive juices that remain pooled at the lower esophageal sphincter area can injure the esophageal tissue, causing bleeding and ulcers within the esophagus and scar tissue formation at the lower end of the esophagus.

This esophageal erosion and ulceration can cause narrowing of the opening around the LES valve and be very painful. Others might not have any clear visual indication of disease of the esophagus; however, they may experience severe symptoms of acid reflux disease and have a very poor quality of life.

Esophageal Strictures

Esophageal strictures are a complication of those who have erosive reflux disease; people with non-erosive reflux disease are not thought to be at risk for strictures. There is no evidence to suggest that erosive reflux disease is a greater risk for cancer development.

Esophageal Cancer

Esophageal adenocarcinoma occurs in a small proportion of people. Recognized risk factors for esophageal cancer include a long history of acid reflux disease with severe symptoms, obesity, and Barrett's esophagus. Medications that act to relax the lower esophageal sphincter muscle may also contribute to increasing the risk of cancer. People felt to be at high risk of developing esophageal cancer need to be monitored regularly by a gastroenterologist.

Did You Know...

A diet low in cereal fiber, fruits, and vegetables is thought to increase the risk of esophageal cancer.

Common Treatments

There are several accepted strategies for treating acid reflux, depending on the severity of the symptoms and associated risk factors.

Over-the-Counter Medications

Over-the-counter medications can neutralize the acid or control the total amount of acid and digestive juices available from the stomach, providing relief from the pain of acid reflux. Controlling stomach acid will decrease the pain of heartburn and indigestion and also reduce the backflow of acid from the stomach, which contributes to the throat discomfort.

Did You Know...

People often begin treating the disease on their own, using a variety of over-the-counter preparations from the pharmacy that are designed to control the action of stomach acid in the esophagus.

There are a number of over-the counter preparations available. Some products, such as calcium carbonate preparations (for example, Tums), are designed to neutralize stomach acid, while other preparations (for example, Zantac, Pepcid) are designed to reduce the total amount of acid and digestive juices available from the stomach. Most people find that these medications provide relief, often for months, and some for many years.

Medical Procedures

Drug Treatment

When over-the-counter preparations can no longer provide complete and predictable relief, it's time to consult your doctor for an assessment and further diagnostic evaluation. Doctors will often prescribe higher doses of agents that will reduce the amount of digestive juices and acid produced by the stomach. If pain relief is inadequate from these agents, then more powerful medications that more precisely target the action of the stomach may be prescribed.

Surgical Intervention

When undertaken on carefully selected patients, surgery can have a very positive influence on quality of life. Conversely, patients who do not meet the appropriate criteria for surgery but move ahead with this intervention may not experience a significant change in quality of life.

Open abdominal or open thoracic are the two procedures traditionally used in surgical treatment. Recently, minimally invasive laparoscopic surgery has become a preferred approach by some. If laparoscopic surgery is chosen, be sure to select a center and a surgeon with significant expertise.

Lifestyle Changes

A balanced lifestyle, featuring regular physical activity, stress management, and a nutritious diet that incorporates well-tolerated foods, is effective not only for treating chronic heartburn but also for preventing this disorder. Begin by adding regular physical activity to your daily routine.

Re-examine your diet to see if you can make any improvements. Eliminating or replacing citrus fruits,

Treatment Protocols

Treatment for chronic heartburn depends upon the severity and the duration of the symptoms. Follow the first program if your symptoms are mild or infrequent, and the second if your symptoms are moderate to severe or frequent.

One: Mild or Infrequent Symptoms

Heartburn
⬇
Mild symptoms less than twice a week
⬇
Respond well to over-the-counter preparations
⬇
Continue with over-the-counter preparations
⬇
Lifestyle modifications: exercise, stress management, diet

Two: Moderate to Severe or Frequent Symptoms

Moderate to severe or frequent symptoms more than twice a week
⬇
Not responding as well to over-the counter preparations
⬇
Arrange for an appointment with your doctor for medical treatment
⬇
Lifestyle modifications: exercise, stress management, diet

tomatoes, carbonated drinks, and alcohol can be a starting point because these products can trigger reflux-like symptoms without necessarily causing reflux. Stress management is another area that will need your attention. Improving your diet and physical activity will help with controlling stress, but don't forget social relationships. Stay connected with family and friends; they are the social networks that will help you with stress management. If cigarettes are still part of your life, work at gradually removing them and control the use of alcohol.

Q: How long will this problem of acid reflux go on?

A: Acid reflux is a very common disorder; it also tends to be a chronic disorder. There are many factors that can lead to the development and continuation of problems with acid reflux. For people who have mild symptoms that occur from time to time, without any significant disruption in their lives, over-the-counter medications and lifestyle modifications are probably adequate to manage problems with acid reflux.

For people who have more severe disease that occurs regularly and interferes with quality of life, it is best to be managed by a doctor who can monitor disease activity. Severe disease tends to be more chronic, meaning that it is not likely to be "cured" but usually can be managed using a combination of medication and lifestyle modifications, including diet.

Case History: Dan

Dan consults the doctor about his reflux symptoms because they are beginning to have a significant impact on his quality of life. His doctor reviews Dan's symptoms and any over-the-counter medications that he has been using for the past couple of years. The doctor asks Dan how he is able to control the pain, what treatments have worked for him in the past, which foods he can tolerate and which foods trigger heartburn. Since certain medications might also aggravate his symptoms, the doctor reviews Dan's use of prescribed medications for other health problems.

After completing the medical history and physical, the doctor suggests that Dan will need a prescription for stronger medications, called H2-blockers, that act to reduce the amount of acid produced by the stomach. If these medications are not effective in providing relief, another group of more powerful agents, called proton pump inhibitors (PPIs), will be prescribed. His doctor indicates that if symptoms persist and worsen, an evaluation by a gastroenterologist might be indicated.

During Dan's medical evaluation, the doctor asks questions about the nutritional quality of his diet, food allergies, alcohol consumption, and weight history. He is particularly interested in looking for potential risk factors for serious disease, so he asks Dan if there has been any evidence of blood loss or anemia and if he has experienced any other pain or difficulty with swallowing. In addition, he inquires about a history of smoking. These are all factors that might be linked to his problems with gastroesophageal reflux.

Dan begins to feel that his chronic heartburn can be managed effectively with medications and lifestyle changes. Perhaps he won't need to see the gastroenterologist after all . . .

(continued, page 48)

CHAPTER 2

What Causes Chronic Heartburn?

Case History: Donna

Donna is a 34-year-old woman who has a 4-year history of heartburn after heavy meals, followed by acid reflux from the stomach, causing a sour taste in her mouth. Recently, her acid reflux symptoms have been increasing, particularly at night. Her doctor has prescribed medication to treat her symptoms and advised Donna to work on modifying her lifestyle. She has an 18-year history of smoking 20 to 25 cigarettes a day. She uses alcohol moderately (30 to 60 mL, 5 days per week), and she drinks five large cups of coffee a day. Over the past 5 years, Donna has gained 45 pounds, which she feels is the result of a stressful job and personal life issues. Her doctor explains that these habits are factors contributing to her chronic heartburn by weakening her lower esophageal sphincter muscle — or LES, to use her doctor's term for this muscle.

The primary physiological cause of acid reflux is a lower esophageal sphincter valve that doesn't work in the way it was meant to — it tends to stay open longer than it should or it closes and opens at the wrong time. The normal tight muscle control of the opening and closing of this valve can be lost due to several factors, including transient muscle relaxations and a hiatus hernia.

Primary Causes of Acid Reflux

Weak lower esophageal sphincter (LES) muscle that does not maintain normal muscle tone and cannot provide a tight barrier between the esophagus and stomach.

Transient LES relaxations (TLESRs) that are inappropriate — not "triggered" by swallowing and different from the typical contraction and relaxation of the LES muscle.

Hiatus hernia that interferes with the normal functioning of the anti-reflux barrier, reducing the effectiveness of the complex interaction between the LES muscle, the diaphragm, and the fibrous tissue ligament that keeps the LES in its place at the "hiatus" in the diaphragm.

LES Muscle Weakness

A defect in the basal LES pressure is thought to be a primary problem that explains gastroesophageal reflux. When the digestive system is working normally, the muscles in the esophagus enable the movement of food through the system. They tightly control the opening and closing of the lower esophageal sphincter valve, with assistance from key nerves located in the region of the stomach and LES, regulating the backward movement, or reflux, of acid, digestive juices, and gas. In a weakened state, this muscle may cause significant problems, resulting in inadequate regulation of the digestive system.

A weakening of the muscle action of the LES increases the risk of recurrent problems as a result of acid and digestive juices refluxing into the esophagus and not being returned into the stomach. These fluids can be very irritating to the tissue of the esophagus, causing the burning pain of heartburn and the sour taste of acid in the throat.

Transient LES Relaxations

The LES muscle can be weakened by transient relaxations (TLESRs). Transient relaxations of the LES are continually occurring within the digestive tract, instigated by the act of swallowing. However, these relaxations are sometimes inappropriate or poorly timed. Unlike its role in triggering "appropriate" LES relaxations, swallowing sometimes does not trigger the transient relaxations of the LES. As a result, the LES opens and closes at the wrong time in the digestive process.

While it is not clear how these inappropriate transient relaxations are triggered within the body, they may be related to the quantity and kind of food we eat. The association of transient relaxations with reflux activity is increased after eating meals and while lying down. Interestingly, a large proportion

Did You Know...

Research has indicated that a full stomach following a meal can act as a trigger to increase transient relaxations, resulting in increased symptoms of reflux. Research has also indicated that as fats and complex starches move into the small bowel from the stomach, there is a delay in emptying the stomach. The emptying of the lower part of the stomach, through the valve mechanism, into the small bowel may also be delayed, causing a slowdown in the process of digestion.

of the population with acid reflux problems describe their symptoms as most obvious after meals, while some experience heartburn and reflux during the night while trying to sleep. Transient relaxations of the LES valve seem to explain the key symptoms of gastroesophageal reflux.

Q: How does food relate to transient lower esophageal sphincter relaxations?

A: Following a meal, a full stomach increases these muscle relaxations, causing increased reflux and increased symptoms. As dietary fats and complex starches move out of the stomach and into the small bowel, they delay emptying of the stomach, thereby causing increased numbers of transient relaxations. Certain types of carbohydrate foods that are not well digested within the large bowel, or colon, have been found to change LES pressure and increase TLESRs in association with acid reflux.

Did You Know...

Meal size and meal composition may have an influence on triggering reflux symptoms. A recent study suggested that certain types of carbohydrate foods that are not digested within the colon could also provide a stimulus to change LES pressure and increase transient LES relaxations in association with acid reflux.

Hiatus Hernia

The lower esophageal sphincter muscle can also be weakened by a hiatus hernia. Hiatus hernia is a very common disorder that results from the movement of the upper part of the stomach above the diaphragm into the chest area. Usually, hiatus hernias are thought to be insignificant clinically. These

Did You Know...

The symptoms of heartburn can be aggravated by feelings of anxiety, fear, and anger. The position of the body, such as lying down and bending forward, can also increase the pain of heartburn.

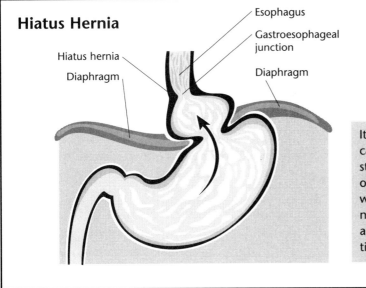

Hiatus Hernia

- Esophagus
- Gastroesophageal junction
- Diaphragm
- Hiatus hernia
- Diaphragm

It's not clear how a hiatus hernia causes reflux of acid from the stomach. Chronic inflammation of the lower esophagus, along with scar tissue, might cause a narrowing of the lower esophagus and weaken the muscle tone of tissue in the LES valve area.

hernias are felt to be the result of a lack of muscle tone in the area of the diaphragm and a lack of muscle tone in the area of the LES valve.

The mechanism by which the hernia might cause reflux of acid from the stomach is unclear. In some cases of acid reflux disease, the development of a hiatus hernia may be the result of chronic inflammation of the lower esophagus, along with scar tissue, that together cause a narrowing of the lower esophagus and weaken the muscle tone of tissue in the LES valve area. This can set the stage for the development of acid reflux. In people with severe symptoms, it has recently been found that the presence of a hiatus hernia results in more severe problems with reflux along with significant esophageal tissue damage.

Other Factors

The changes in functioning of the LES muscle that cause acid reflux are influenced by many other factors that differ from one person to another.

Smoking and Alcohol

For decades, those with symptoms of acid reflux have been advised to discontinue smoking and to avoid alcohol. Alcohol and cigarettes have been found to change the peristaltic movement of muscle throughout the esophagus and to reduce the muscle tone at the lower end of the esophagus at the LES.

Fatty Foods

Certain foods can also aggravate heartburn. Meals that are higher in fat content might contribute to decreasing muscle tone of the LES. High-fat meals are emptied from the stomach more slowly than low-fat meals, which may play a role in decreasing the LES muscle tone. Slower emptying of the stomach may contribute to inappropriate relaxation of the LES, enabling acid reflux to continue.

Troublesome Foods

Some foods have been identified as being "troublesome" factors in acid reflux, relaxing the LES valve or irritating the esophageal tissue.

Troublesome Foods

Foods that relax the LES valve	Foods that can irritate esophageal tissue
Chocolate	Citrus juices and citrus products
Caffeine-containing foods/beverages	Tomato products
Alcohol	Coffee
Mint	Spirits
Fat	
Onions	
Garlic	
Spices	

Troublesome Medications

Some medications have been identified as being "troublesome" factors in acid reflux, relaxing the LES valve or delaying the emptying of the stomach.

Troublesome Medications

Medications that relax the LES valve	Medications that can delay stomach emptying
Alpha-adrenergic blockers	Anticholinergic agents
Anticholinergic agents	Narcotic analgesics
Benzodiazepines	
Beta2 agonists	
Calcium channel blockers	
Dopamine	
Estrogen	
Narcotic analgesics	
Nicotine	
Nitrates	
Progesterone	
Prostaglandins	
Theophylline	
Tricyclic antidepressants	

Overweight and Obesity

Traditionally, obesity has been considered to be a factor in causing acid reflux, the result of obese abdominal tissue compressing the stomach area. The pressure exerted on the stomach may contribute to weakening of the LES valve, allowing acid and digestive juices to back up into the esophagus. When obese people with acid reflux problems lose weight, they often find that problems with heartburn and reflux significantly improve.

Case History: David

David is a 62-year-old man with a long history of problems with heartburn and acid reflux, often with pain behind the breastbone that is felt in his back. Throughout the day, he has heartburn that he treats with antacid medication. About 25 years ago, David was told that he had a hiatus hernia. Recently, he has noticed that his voice is hoarse. He is also having problems swallowing solid foods.

He thinks that he has lost weight over the last month as a result of his problems with swallowing.

David's history suggests that his disease has been progressing, despite his regular use of over-the-counter medications. It is time for him to arrange an appointment with his doctor to be evaluated and closely monitored for weight and disease activity.

CHAPTER 3

Who Is at Risk of Developing Chronic Heartburn?

Case History: Elaine

Elaine is 32 and midway through her first pregnancy. She had been feeling well and progressing as expected with her pregnancy, but recently, digestive tract problems have begun to interfere with her life. Elaine has never been bothered by stomach problems before, so when she begins to experience a burning pain behind her breastbone and an acid taste in her mouth that are associated with eating, she becomes rather concerned. Her doctor indicates that her symptoms suggest gastroesophageal reflux.

Although chronic heartburn may afflict us at any time during our lives, pregnant women, infants, children, the elderly, and the overweight and obese are at greatest risk of developing reflux disease, though symptoms and their severity may vary. During pregnancy, a significant proportion of women experience problems with acid reflux. Infants, children, and adolescents also experience varying degrees of acid reflux. Toward the end of life, the elderly experience an overall decrease in muscle tone throughout the body, making them vulnerable to acid reflux problems, often associated with motility changes. Obesity, at any age, is an important risk factor for the development of chronic heartburn and acid reflux disease.

Pregnancy

Acid reflux is a common occurrence during pregnancy, affecting anywhere from one-third to two-thirds of all women. The problem usually begins several months into the pregnancy and resolves shortly after delivery of the baby. As the pregnancy progresses, women tend to have increasing problems with heartburn.

Causes

The primary cause of the problem is a decrease in muscle tone of the lower esophageal sphincter (LES).

Stomach Pressure

The primary reason for the decrease in muscle tone of the LES may be the pressure of the growing baby pushing against the stomach and exerting enough pressure within the stomach to weaken the LES muscle. Abdominal obesity is thought to weaken the LES valve in this way, so perhaps a growing baby will exert a similar mechanical obstruction to the stomach and also weaken the LES valve mechanism. The growing baby does exert pressure against and within the stomach, but it is not clear if this is the cause of reflux problems during pregnancy. Other factors likely explain how acid reflux problems begin and progress through pregnancy.

Hormones

The key hormones of pregnancy, progesterone and estrogen, have been found to be the primary factors that bring on the symptoms of gastroesophageal reflux. Progesterone, when working in conjunction with estrogen, causes a decrease of pressure in the LES valve, causing a weakening of muscle tone. A partially open valve allows acidic digestive juices to back up into the esophagus. The result is heartburn.

Motility

Changes in motility, the muscle action that moves food through the digestive tract, also contribute to reflux problems.

Q: How does the doctor diagnose this problem during pregnancy?

A: Symptoms of heartburn associated with meals during pregnancy are a common finding. Rather than testing for acid reflux disease, doctors use clinical judgment and treat the person's symptoms.

Treatment Options

The goal of therapy is to try to minimize symptoms of acid reflux. Medications are not usually used during pregnancy unless absolutely necessary. Treatment is focused on lifestyle modifications, though antacids and barrier treatments have proven to be effective in some cases.

Lifestyle Modifications

- Eating frequent, small meals that are not rich in food sources of fat
- Avoiding foods that may cause heartburn
- Avoiding food or fluids late at night or shortly before going to bed
- Avoiding bending forward
- Raising the head of the bed so gravity will maintain acidic digestive juices within the stomach, thereby decreasing problems with heartburn

Antacids

Antacids are used to relieve mild symptoms of heartburn and acid reflux in people with gastroesophageal reflux (GER) or GERD. They act to neutralize stomach acids, using preparations containing calcium, magnesium, or aluminum, along with bicarbonate or hydroxide.

If medications are used during pregnancy, those that are well tolerated tend to be calcium/magnesium-based antacid preparations.

Classical antacid products

- Alka-Seltzer
- Maalox
- Mylanta
- Pepto-Bismol
- Rolaids
- Riopan
- Tums

Typical barrier agents

- Sulcrate (sucralfate)
- Gaviscon products: Gaviscon Acid Relief; Gaviscon Heartburn Relief

---

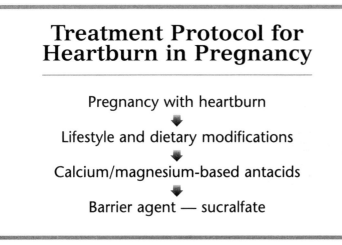

Treatment Protocol for Heartburn in Pregnancy

Pregnancy with heartburn
⬇
Lifestyle and dietary modifications
⬇
Calcium/magnesium-based antacids
⬇
Barrier agent — sucralfate

Barrier Agents

Barrier agents act as a protective layer that minimizes or separates the action of stomach acid from the delicate tissue of the esophagus, thereby providing control of the reflux of stomach acid into the esophagus.

Infancy

Stomach acid reflux is very common in about 50% of infants as a result of the immaturity of the digestive system. The movement of food and fluids through the esophagus and stomach often occurs in an unorganized and unregulated way. Sometimes it moves through the system as expected, while other times it may back up into the esophagus and up into the mouth. In most cases, acid reflux in infants gradually resolves over time.

The LES valve often tends to relax in a way that is not related to swallowing in infants who have an immature digestive tract. Short-term use of medications that enhance the movement of food through the digestive system (motility agents) is sometimes used to decrease problems with reflux. Once children are able to tolerate solid foods, as well as sit up on their own and walk, problems of acid reflux tend to disappear in most cases.

Case History: Erin

Since birth, Erin has had problems with frequent spitting up or regurgitation and vomiting, associated with feeding. She is now a year old. Her mother has tried to assist Erin by providing thickened feedings and positioning her to enable solids and fluids to move readily into the stomach. These approaches have helped, but she still has times when her mom's assistance is not quite enough to control her problems with vomiting associated with food intake. When she takes fluids that are not thickened, such as juice and water, she has problems with the fluid backing up into her mouth, rather than moving into her stomach and then progressing through the digestive system.

Childhood

Problems with gastroesophageal reflux are not uncommon in children. As with other cases of acid reflux, the primary cause of the problem is a decrease in muscle tone of the lower esophageal sphincter.

A child's problem with acid reflux might be the result of a genetic predisposition to having an LES muscle that does not function optimally. Other factors to consider when evaluating this problem are an increase in body weight, which might interfere with the normal functioning of the LES valve. Poor diet may also be a factor. Lack of physical activity, important in helping to tone muscles within the body, and possibly undiagnosed stress, might be further factors.

Treating Acid Reflux in Infants and Children

- Thicken feedings for infants
- Eat frequent small meals
- Manage weight for overweight and obese children
- Avoid aggravating foods:
  - foods high in fat
  - foods high in acid (citrus, tomato, carbonated drinks)
  - coffee
  - chocolate
- Avoid food between dinner and bedtime
- Avoid tight-fitting clothing
- Position body to prevent reflux: upright or prone positions

Did You Know...

Reflux does not tend to persist after age 2. However, the first 2 years of life can be incredibly frustrating for parents who have a child with severe reflux problems. In severe cases, regurgitation and vomiting can result in fluid imbalance and the risk of dehydration. The infant might be incredibly hungry but not be able to retain a great deal of fluid and food due to a disordered movement of food and fluids through an immature digestive tract.

Case History: Eric

Eric is an anxious 10-year-old boy who has been experiencing problems with heartburn and a taste of acid in the back of his throat, associated with food intake, over the past year. His pediatrician has been managing his condition with antacid preparations, which have helped somewhat; however, he is now experiencing pain during the night, which is interfering with his getting adequate sleep. Eric has never been physically active; he enjoys watching television and using his computer, rather than participating in sports. His weight has been above normal for the past 3 years, which his mother says is the result of poor food choices.

The Elderly

The prevalence of chronic heartburn and acid reflux in the elderly has been increasing over the past several years. While it is not clear why this is occurring, there are a number of factors that might contribute to the problem. With aging, changes occur in the muscular movement (peristaltic waves) within the esophagus. Changes in the function of the LES valve have also been found in the elderly. Movement of food through the digestive tract may be slower, with the result that chances of acid refluxing from the stomach into the esophagus might be increased. Individuals who are on multiple medications for other health problems often find that symptoms of acid reflux are aggravated as a result of tissue injury to the esophagus, changes in the action of the LES valve, or medications being taken.

Relapse in the disease is common once medications for acid reflux are discontinued. The need for constant medication, as well as problems of relapse when medications are discontinued, can further interfere with the quality of life for the elderly population.

Case History: Edward

Edward is a 75-year-old gentleman who has had a long history of gastroesophageal reflux. His main complaints over the years have been heartburn and acid reflux, felt and tasted in his throat, often associated with meals. He frequently feels pain that radiates to his back, especially during the night, which disturbs his sleep. More recently, Edward has been experiencing problems with swallowing, regurgitation of meals, and sometimes vomiting associated with meals. His weight has decreased by 10 pounds in the past 4 months.

Many medications have been used in the past to treat his problem, but recently they have not been as effective in controlling pain. His symptoms are now significantly interfering with his quality of life.

Overweight and Obesity

Research studies indicate that people with a weight problem may have more problems with acid reflux than people at a normal weight. In fact, several recent studies have documented a clear association among overweight and obesity, esophageal erosions, and symptoms of gastroesophageal reflux disease. Abdominal obesity is felt to increase the pressure around the stomach, potentially weakening the lower esophageal sphincter valve, allowing acid and digestive juices to back up into the esophagus. Symptoms of acid reflux have been found to decrease with loss of body weight.

Any person with significant weight problems is capable of developing complications of gastroesophageal reflux disease. Research suggests that it depends on how long the person has been experiencing symptoms. People over age 60 with a long history of symptoms are at greater risk of developing complications. So it's important to monitor changes in weight in the elderly.

Case History: Ellen

Ellen has experienced progressive weight gain over the past few years. The mother of three young children, she has a hectic lifestyle, working at a full-time position as an office assistant. The weight gained with each pregnancy was only partially lost, so over the past 8 years she has gained about 100 lbs (45 kg). She has not been successful at losing the weight, despite trying various diet regimens. During the past 3 years she has been experiencing increasing problems with reflux disease, requiring prescribed medications to control the heartburn and acid reflux.

Ellen's increase in weight over the past few years may be an important contributor to the symptoms of acid reflux that she is experiencing. She reports that acid reflux is particularly noticeable following heavy meals. Recently, she has noted that her symptoms are becoming more troublesome during the night.

CHAPTER 4

When Do You Need to See Your Doctor?

Case History: Sandra

Sandra is a 40-year-old woman with more than 10 years of problems with severe heartburn and acid reflux into her throat that occurs after meals, when she leans forward, and while she is lying in bed. Her doctor has been prescribing medication (proton pump inhibitors) at intervals during the past few years, which used to provide relief of Sandra's symptoms. Recently, she has found that she no longer has the same control of her symptoms.

She consulted a gastroenterologist recently who did endoscopic studies, using a gastroscope, to evaluate the tissue of her esophagus and stomach so he could determine whether she had complicating problems that would explain her symptoms. He reassured her that he found nothing of concern in the examination.

Sandra has a type of acid reflux that shows no evidence of serious disease on endoscopy studies. The description of her disease would be endoscopy-negative gastroesophageal reflux that shows no tissue erosion of the esophagus. While Sandra was relieved that no serious complications were discovered, she is frustrated that her current experience with pain is still interfering with her quality of life.

Did You Know...

Well-designed and validated questionnaires on quality of life have been frequently used over the past several years to evaluate how people are coping with this frustrating and painful disorder.

As providers of primary care, family physicians are the logical first place to turn for advice on how to approach acid reflux disease that is not readily responding to over-the-counter therapy. To evaluate your symptoms, the doctor will conduct a physical examination and take a medical history, including use of over-the-counter medications. Recent work is being done on the use of symptom-focused questionnaires to enable patients to describe how symptoms of acid reflux disease intrude on their quality of life. Increasingly, it is felt that recognizing people's feelings about what they are experiencing is crucial to guiding treatment approaches and decisions.

Quality of Life
Gastrointestinal Short Form Questionnaire (GSFQ)

Instructions
Answer each question by checking one box. If you are unsure about how to answer a question, please give the best answer you can. These questions are about how stomach problems have affected you during the past week.

How much of the time during the past week	All of the time	Most of the time	Some of the time	A little of the time	None of the time
Score (marks):	(4)	(3)	(2)	(1)	(0)
1. Have you had pain or discomfort in the upper abdomen, such as burning, bloating or fullness?	___	___	___	___	___
2. Have you had pain or discomfort in the area of the breast bone, such as heartburn, fullness, or sensation of blockage?	___	___	___	___	___
3. Have you been limited in eating a normal meal or in your choice of foods or beverages because of your stomach problems?	___	___	___	___	___
4. Do you experience a rising, spreading, burning sensation behind your breastbone (heartburn)?	___	___	___	___	___

5. During the past week, have your normal daily activities been affected by your heartburn?
❑ No
❑ Yes

If yes, how many days of daily activities have been affected during the past week?

Score (1 mark per day): _____(days)

6. During the past week, has your sleep been disturbed because of your heartburn?
❑ No
❑ Yes

If yes, how many nights of sleep have been disturbed during the past week?

Score (1 mark per night): _____(nights)

Total Score (Questions 1–6): _____

Scoring System
The first 4 questions reflect frequency of symptoms and are scored from 0–4. The last 2 questions are an indication of quality of life: they are scored as 1 mark for each day that symptoms of acid reflux/GERD interfere with quality of life. If your total score is:

0–2: Symptoms are **mild**: occasional antacids needed.

3–6: Symptoms are **moderate**: may respond to intermittent use of over-the-counter antacids on a more regular basis, or to over-the-counter H2-RA medications (Zantac, Pepcid, etc.).

7–15: Symptoms are **severe**: may respond to the regular use of over-the-counter H2-RAs, but you should consider consulting your physician.

16–30: Symptoms are **very severe**: consult your physician; you may be given a prescription for a proton pump inhibitor (PPI).

Adapted by permission from Paré P, Meyer F, Armstrong D, Pyzyk M, Pericak D, Goeree R. Validation of the GSFQ, a self-administered symptom frequency questionnaire for patients with gastroesophageal reflux disease. Can J Gastroenterol 2003;17(5):307–12.

Diagnosis

In North America, the standard medical practice for diagnosing gastroesophageal reflux disease is based on the symptoms described by the patient. Typically, when a patient visits the doctor and describes symptoms of heartburn and possibly acid reflux, the patient will be treated with over-the-counter medications to control the symptoms, usually without additional diagnostic investigations.

However, sometimes the doctor may suggest that a more detailed diagnostic workup be completed before prescribing medications, depending on the findings from the history and the physical exam, as well as a consideration of the nature and severity of any symptoms — particularly if there are any "red flags" suggesting unusual findings.

Presumptive Diagnosis

When patients describe the typical symptoms of heartburn and acid reflux into the throat, the doctor makes a presumptive diagnosis. Doctors tend to make a "presumptive diagnosis" of GERD when the history and physical findings point to the likelihood of GERD.

If the patient has an improvement in symptoms when using the medications designed to treat acid reflux disease, it is presumed that the diagnosis is in fact accurate.

Endoscopy and Gastroscopy

If there is a change in symptoms or there are problems in managing the disease, the primary care physician may refer patients to a gastroenterologist, who will then do an endoscopic procedure to evaluate the tissue of the esophagus, looking for changes that might explain the patient's symptoms.

To check for serious disease progression and complications, your doctor may request an endoscopy or gastroscopy. The term "endoscope" or "endoscopy" is a general one that indicates that a camera will be used to view the *interior* of the digestive tract. It might be from the top end or the bottom end of the digestive tract. The term "gastroscope" or "gastroscopy" indicates that the scope used will be introduced via the mouth, studying the area from the mouth through the esophagus to the stomach.

Q: What is the procedure for an endoscopy or gastroscopy?

A: Gastroscopy and endoscopy studies are usually undertaken in an endoscopy unit of a hospital or clinic. Usually a muscle relaxant is given to patients to decrease anxiety and promote relaxation. The procedure involves passing a long thin rubber-type tube, mounted with powerful camera lenses, through the mouth and down into the esophagus, through the lower esophageal sphincter valve, and into the stomach. The procedure itself happens quite quickly, with the doctor moving the tube through the upper part of the digestive tract, carefully watching for tissue changes that might signify problems, and obtaining tissue biopsies if necessary.

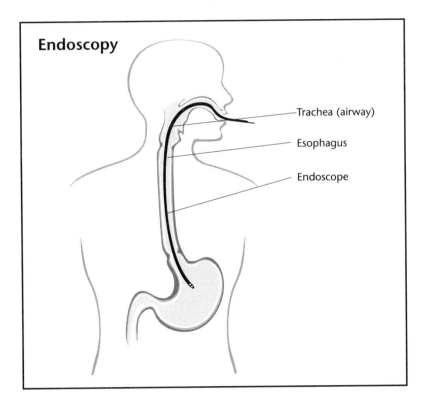

Endoscopy

Trachea (airway)

Esophagus

Endoscope

These diagnostic procedures are not done on everybody who has symptoms of acid reflux disease, and the majority of people will not have any disease noted in the esophagus or stomach when endoscopy studies are done. However, when symptoms persist or fail to respond to over-the-counter and prescribed drugs, these procedures can be informative and preventive.

Case History: Sam

Sam is a 59-year-old man who has a 10-year history of acid reflux disease that has responded well to proton pump inhibitor medications (PPIs) in the past. Recently, he lost 10 pounds unintentionally and has experienced some problems with swallowing solid foods, some episodes of vomiting, and blood loss. His most recent blood test showed a new finding of anemia. Sam's doctor explained that these new symptoms indicate that Sam's disease has changed, and referred him to a gastroenterologist, who evaluated Sam's esophagus and stomach with endoscopy studies. Changes in the tissue of the esophagus were discovered, indicating that Barrett's esophagus was present.

Barrett's esophagus is a disorder indicating that normal esophageal tissue at the level of the lower esophageal sphincter has been replaced with a different kind of tissue that might be at risk of converting to cancer in the future. As Sam's doctor emphasizes, this is only a possibility, not a certainty. When people are diagnosed with Barrett's esophagus, a gastroenterologist watches for further tissue changes and closely monitors them with regular endoscopy studies.

Case History: Scott

Scott is a 51-year-old man who has experienced problems with acid reflux for the past 5 years, with chronic heartburn in his chest and reflux into his throat. The pain has been increasing. Scott has had some difficulties swallowing food, which has interfered with his usual dietary intake. His doctor referred him to a gastroenterologist, who decided that it was time to view his upper digestive tract, using an endoscope. The endoscopy studies indicated that the esophagus had erosions, which are small tears within the esophageal tissue. The esophageal tears are likely the source of Scott's increased pain.

Scott's gastroenterologist explains that his acid reflux disease is complicated by the tissue erosions. The breakdown of tissue in the esophagus will possibly be further aggravated by acid being refluxed back from the stomach into the esophagus, bathing the raw open tears present within the esophageal tissue. Because the tears are visible through the endoscope, it will be easier to monitor whether medications used to treat the acid reflux disease are able to heal the erosions, using follow-up endoscopy when necessary.

Only a qualified physician, who has the expertise to evaluate information from the history and physical examination, can make the decision to do endoscopic procedures.

Differential Diagnosis

Symptoms that appear to be typical for acid reflux disease may indicate other disease states. Your doctor might run additional tests if your symptoms resemble the associated symptoms of other disorders or diseases. Other conditions with symptoms similar to GERD include inflammations of the esophagus as a result of fungal or viral infections, Crohn's disease of the esophagus, medications that can irritate the esophageal tissue, peptic ulcers within the stomach, and perhaps heart disease.

Talk to your doctor about other disorders that might be present. Sometimes presenting symptoms of a disorder resemble acid reflux disease in many ways, but have additional features that are not part of the constellation of gastroesophageal reflux.

Heart Disease

For some people, the experience of heartburn, with severe pain in the chest area behind the breastbone, resembles the pain of a heart attack. If there is concern about a potential heart attack, an EKG can be arranged to evaluate this risk.

Depression and Stress

Psychosocial stressors are frequently associated with aggravation of disorders of the gastrointestinal tract. Emotional disturbances have been found to directly influence the motility of the esophagus. Chest pain that is not the result of heart disease has also been associated with feelings of anxiety and symptoms of depression.

Adverse Reactions to Medications

Other medications may cause significant problems that have similar symptoms to acid reflux disease. Be sure to discuss with your doctor all medications being taken.

Pill-induced ulceration of the esophagus can also occur as the result of consuming medications with insufficient fluid. The medication begins to dissolve within the esophageal tissue and, in some cases, can cause significant tissue irritation.

Did You Know...

The experience of heartburn, with severe pain in the chest area behind the breastbone, can resemble the pain of a heart attack. If you experience new-onset chest pain, it is important to have your doctor evaluate whether the pain is due to heart problems or esophageal problems.

Did You Know...

A recent study evaluating the influence of life stress on symptoms of heartburn indicated that major life stressors, as opposed to minor life events or mood changes, are what influence the severity of heartburn. It is possible that prolonged stress may involve psychological as well as physiological mechanisms that exacerbate symptoms of heartburn.

Certain antibiotics, antiviral agents, and non-steroidal anti-inflammatory medications can cause significant problems. The problem can be resolved by ensuring that adequate water is taken with medications to enable them to enter the stomach, where appropriate breakdown can occur.

Bisphosphonate medications, a class of drugs used to prevent the resorption of bone, have been identified as a source of esophageal injury. Erosive esophagitis can occur in a small proportion of patients as a result of this class of medication. Be sure to take this drug when in an upright position with adequate fluid to enable entry into the stomach.

Esophageal Dysmotility

Dysmotility of the esophagus implies that the peristaltic contractions that move food and fluids between the mouth and the stomach are not synchronized. Motility studies are used to evaluate patients with symptoms of dysphagia that is not associated with inflammation or strictures to determine the source of the disordered peristaltic contractions.

Abnormalities in esophageal motility are classified into four main areas:

- Esophageal hypercontractility — may be secondary to GERD
- Esophageal hypocontractility — may be secondary to GERD
- Uncoordinated esophageal contractions — examples include diffuse esophagospasm or "nutcracker" esophagus
- Inadequate relaxation of the LES sphincter — for example, achalasia

Manometric studies are used to identify which abnormalities predominate in esophageal motility. Once the diagnosis is clarified, treatment planning can progress.

Esophageal Ulcer Disease

Ulcer disease tends to be rare within the esophagus. When it does occur, it can be the result of a number of disorders linked with the immune system, including autoimmune disorders, associated genetically inherited disorders, esophageal carcinomas, and associated immune system reactions to fungal or viral infections. In addition, there are skin diseases that are associated with involvement of the esophagus. Endoscopy evaluation will clarify the source of the problem.

Immune System Compromise

Infections within the esophagus are not common in healthy individuals. However, when there is compromise of the immune system, a variety of infections are possible. Candida is the most common source of infection, associated with malnutrition, diabetes, or use of several antibiotics and steroid medications.

Achalasia

Achalasia is an esophageal problem that involves a lack of peristalsis in the esophageal body, between the upper and lower esophageal sphincters, along with an inability of the LES to relax normally. The tight LES muscle acts like a point of obstruction that needs to be treated. The key symptoms include problems with swallowing solids and liquids, regurgitation of undigested food and excessive saliva, chest pain around the area of the breastbone, heartburn that does not follow meals, and weight loss. Patients often experience problems for several years, adapting to the slowly progressive nature of achalasia before consulting a physician.

Treatment is focused on managing symptoms and preventing complications. The primary goal is to reduce the pressure of the LES valve by taking steps to relax the muscle, thereby enabling food and fluid to pass through the esophagus into the stomach.

Zollinger-Ellison Syndrome (ZES)

ZES is a rare condition involving various parts of the digestive system, causing tumors in the duodenum and pancreas, as well as ulcers in the stomach and the duodenum. The tumors secrete a hormone called gastrin that stimulates the stomach to produce more acid than normal.

Other Diagnostic Studies

Sometimes additional studies may be undertaken in an attempt to more clearly understand the severity of the disease or to provide information that can assist with improving the medical therapy being offered. These include ambulatory pH monitoring to evaluate the amount and presence of acid in the esophagus; the proton pump inhibitor study to evaluate whether this class of medications will quickly resolve

Did You Know...

Patients diagnosed with HIV/AIDS have often been noted to have large, deep ulcers of the esophagus. Candida infection is often present as well. Prednisone has been used to manage this type of ulcer disease.

symptoms of acid reflux disease; and the acid perfusion study to determine whether an increase in the sensitivity of the esophagus is causing the heartburn or pain within the chest.

Ambulatory pH Monitoring

This test is sometimes used to diagnose the presence of excess acid within the esophagus in patients receiving standard medical therapy, but who are still having problems with inadequate control of symptoms. A pH electrode, used to measure acid, is connected to a data collector introduced through the mouth into the lower end of the esophagus. This test allows symptoms to be identified and measures acid reflux activity. The frequency and duration can also be measured, giving a clearer idea of how symptoms of acid reflux disease relate to the presence of acid in the lower esophagus.

Proton Pump Inhibitor (PPI) Test

This test involves measuring the response of people suspected of having acid reflux disease to high doses of PPI medication over a short interval. The test is considered positive if there is an improvement of about 50% to 75% in the patient's symptoms with the use of PPI medications.

Acid Perfusion Test (Bernstein Test)

This test involves administering a salt solution and then a chemical acid solution into the esophagus to evaluate if the patient develops pain, heartburn, or other symptoms of acid reflux disease when the acid solution is introduced. It is usually done at the same time as esophageal manometry.

Esophageal Manometry

This test gives an indication of how effectively the muscles of the esophagus and LES valve are working in patients diagnosed with acid reflux disease. People with this disease commonly have a delay in the movement of food through the esophagus and into the stomach. This test gives information about how the pressure of the LES valve and the transient LES relaxations (TLESRs) contribute to the reflux of acid from the stomach into the esophagus, as well as how competent the LES valve is at clearing acid back into the stomach.

Q: Does *Helicobacter pylori (H. pylori)* have anything to do with acid reflux disease?

A: *Helicobacter pylori* is a bacterium that sometimes lives in the stomach, where it causes an inflammatory reaction called gastritis. As it takes up residence in the stomach, *H. pylori* breaks down the thick protective mucus layer of the stomach, which then allows the bacteria and stomach acid to move into the more sensitive layers of tissue, causing a painful inflammatory reaction within the stomach. *H. pylori* is diagnosed by several studies that might involve blood, breath, stool, tissue, or saliva samples. The most common test uses blood, where tests for antibodies to *H. pylori* are evaluated.

There is no evidence to suggest that *H. pylori* causes any of the symptoms of acid reflux. To the contrary, the bacteria may decrease the secretion of acid in the stomach in some people, which suggests that bacteria might be helpful in decreasing the symptoms of acid reflux. The presence of *H. pylori* in the stomach does not interfere with the treatment of GERD. However, if long-term therapy with proton pump inhibitors (PPIs) is required, it is best to eradicate the bacteria, as the *H. pylori* (with or without concurrent PPI therapy) may eventually lead to pre-cancerous changes to the stomach tissue. Triple drug therapy, taken over one or two weeks, is an effective treatment used to destroy the bacteria.

Prognosis

Short-Term

The primary short-term goal is to treat heartburn and acid reflux adequately to promote one's quality of life. The symptoms of heartburn and acid reflux may be mild in some, while in others symptoms might be severe and incapacitating, interfering with one's quality of life. Monitoring patients with standardized questionnaires that identify quality of life factors is increasingly being used to enable people to evaluate how well all types of therapy are meeting their needs.

Did You Know...

Not everybody responds well to medicinal therapy, so it is important to include lifestyle modifications in addition to pharmaceutical support for this disease.

Long-Term

The primary long-term goal is to promote the healing of tissue to reduce the risk of complications, such as the formation of esophageal strictures, which are areas of narrowing within the esophagus that interfere with the movement of food through the esophagus and into the stomach. Prevention of esophageal cancer is another long-term goal.

Complications

The prevalence of complications for this disorder is actually very low. Complications are more likely to develop with erosive reflux disease, which is less prevalent than acid reflux disease. The majority of people with reflux disease have non-erosive disease, which is not thought to develop esophageal tears, ulcers, and fistulas.

Quality of Life

Poor quality of life is a significant problem for many people who experience regular chronic heartburn symptoms that do not respond well to standard therapy. Reflux disease can be unpredictable, can turn your life upside down when least expected, and can have an impact on your productivity and enjoyment of life.

The complication of erosive disease can be extremely painful, though this population is more likely to respond positively and quickly to proton pump inhibitor (PPI) medications that heal inflamed and ulcerated tissue, improving quality of life. Even though pain might be severe with a relapse, knowledge that the PPI medication has worked in the past and is likely to work in the future can be very reassuring.

However, a significant proportion of people with non-erosive reflux disease do not respond so positively to PPI medications, for reasons that are not clearly understood. Quality of life can be a major issue for some with non-erosive disease. Gastroscopy studies tend to be negative, with no evidence of tissue involvement. If PPI treatments do not significantly improve the pain of heartburn, the inability to control the disorder can be frustrating, contributing to a poor quality of life.

Did You Know...

Primary risk factors for the development of esophageal cancer include the length of time that acid reflux has been experienced, signs of Barrett's esophagus, and obesity. Dietary choices and medications that relax the LES may also contribute to the increased incidence of esophageal cancer in Western nations.

Acid Reflux Disease Treatments

CHAPTER 5

Drug Treatments

Case History: Dan

Dan has found that the pain he has been experiencing with heartburn has become increasingly severe, and he feels that overall his symptoms of GERD are no longer being controlled using his current approach to treatment. His use of over-the-counter antacids and low-dose H2-RA medication is not nearly as effective as it was in the past. His doctor suggests that prescribed proton pump inhibitors (PPIs) are the best choice to attempt to control his disease.

Both over-the-counter (OTC) and prescriptions drugs have been proven to be very effective in treating the symptoms of chronic heartburn and acid reflux disease. Prokinetic agents, sensory modulators, and some herbal remedies can also offer relief.

Over-the-Counter (OTC) Preparations

There are a number of preparations that are helpful in treating mild cases of acid reflux or gastroesophageal reflux. The product categories are antacids, alginates, and low-dose histamine-2 receptor antagonists (H2-RAs). These preparations are readily available without a prescription, so they tend to be the first choice in treatment for acid reflux when people are managing symptoms on their own.

Popular Antacids

- Alka-Seltzer
- Maalox
- Mylanta
- Pepto-Bismol
- Rolaids
- Riopan
- Tums

Antacids

Antacids are used to relieve mild symptoms of heartburn and acid reflux. They act to neutralize stomach acids, using preparations containing calcium, magnesium, or aluminum, along with bicarbonate or hydroxide.

Alginates

Alginic acid or alginate is extracted from seaweed, refined, and then added to antacid products. The unique properties of alginate products enable the separation of stomach acid from the esophagus, via a "floating bridge of foam," made up of sodium alginate. This "foam" provides control of the reflux of stomach acid into the esophagus.

Barrier Agents

Barrier agents are another class of non-prescription medications that tend to be well tolerated. They act locally on the esophageal and gastric tissue to protect the tissue mucosa from being irritated by acidic products, such as stomach juices and chemicals or drugs that might be consumed.

Low-Dose Histamine-2 Receptor Antagonists (H2-RAs)

H2-RAs, also known as H2 blockers, are a class of medications that prevent the production of acid by the stomach. Specifically, these drugs prevent the chemical transmitter histamine from stimulating the parietal cell that releases hydrochloric acid into the stomach cavity, or lumen. Low-dose preparations can be used without a prescription for the treatment of acid reflux. Unfortunately, the effect of H2-RAs diminishes with time and is overcome readily by the effect of food.

Popular Alginates

- Gaviscon Products: Gaviscon Acid Relief; Gaviscon Heartburn Relief

---

Popular Barrier Agents

- Sulcrate (sucralfate)

Low-Dose Histamine-2 Receptor Antagonists (H2-RAs)

- Cimetidine (Tagamet)
- Ranitidine (Zantac)
- Famotidine (Pepcid)
- Nizatidine (Axid)

Prescription Medications

When acid reflux becomes an ongoing problem that impinges on your quality of life, requiring treatment on a regular basis, your doctor will need to develop a plan of care to meet your specific needs. Your doctor is your guide on how to manage acid reflux disease using medications.

Prescription medications, designed to rapidly turn off acid production from the stomach, may be used to provide rapid control of the symptoms. The doctor may prescribe medications that are stronger than those available over the counter.

There are two classes of medications that would be considered: histamine-2 receptor antagonists (H2-RA) blockers

---

Did You Know...

Alginates are well tolerated during pregnancy, as are barrier agents that act to protect esophageal tissue. They can be used if other treatments are not proving effective.

Proton Pump Inhibitors (PPIs)

- Esomeprazole (Nexium)
- Lansoprazole (Prevacid)
- Omeprazole (Losec/ Prilosec)
- Pantoprazole (Pantoloc)
- Rabeprazole (Pariet/ Aciphex)

Did You Know...

Proton pump inhibitors tend to be the medication of choice for treating acid reflux disease.

in a stronger dose to treat disease that is moderately severe; and proton pump inhibitors (PPIs), which are more powerful agents than H2 blockers, to reduce acid secretion.

Proton Pump Inhibitors (PPIs)

Proton pump inhibitors are the most effective medication for the treatment of acid reflux disease. Like H2 blockers, they are designed to prevent the secretion of acid by the proton pump within the stomach; however, the action of PPIs is much more powerful, causing an irreversible blockage of the proton pump in the stomach. This lasts for 2 to 3 days, until the parietal cell replaces the blocked pumps with new, functioning pumps.

People with frequent "flares" of disease and severe symptoms are often managed on long-term PPIs. Those with milder disease are often able to reduce the dose or discontinue medications for a period of time. For example, they might be prescribed a PPI medication initially, then be able to "step down" to a lower dose, even to an H2 blocker, and perhaps be able to discontinue medical therapy until a relapse of symptoms in the future.

Medication prescribed "on demand" is how some physicians manage patients who might have intermittent symptoms that require medication some of the time. Medication will be stopped during times when symptoms are well controlled, and then restarted to treat symptoms.

Although PPI medications have been recognized as revolutionary in targeting the primary source of the problem in reflux disease, for reasons unknown they do not work for everybody with the disease. About one-third of people with non-erosive or endoscopy-negative reflux disease do not respond to the PPI medications.

Q: When is it time to turn to your doctor for assistance?

A: When symptoms become increasingly severe, enough to interfere with usual daily activities and require the regular use of over-the-counter medication — it's time to consult your doctor! A decrease in the response to over-the-counter medications, along with more severe symptoms of acid reflux, suggest that medical advice is required.

Other Pharmacologic Agents

Prokinetic Agents

Prokinetic agents are medications designed to increase the pressure of the lower esophageal sphincter valve, which facilitates the emptying of the stomach into the small bowel. These agents may have various effects on the digestive system:

- Improve esophageal transit, or the speed at which food and fluids move through the digestive tract.
- Improve esophageal clearance of refluxed acid.
- Increase LES pressure, thereby reducing problems with reflux.
- Increase the rate of emptying of contents of the stomach into the small bowel, decreasing the risk of reflux.
- Affect other symptoms that are not related to reflux — for example, decrease problems with bloating.
- Reduce problems with constipation through the increased rate of clearance of foods and fluids through the digestive system.

Sensory Modulators

Sensory modulators include anti-anxiety and antidepressant medications. Psychosocial stressors frequently have a significant influence on the functioning of the gastrointestinal tract. The use of anti-anxiety drugs or antidepressants might be indicated in some individuals who are troubled by digestive disease symptoms that do not respond to standard anti-reflux therapy. However, tricyclic antidepressants have been identified as being capable of relaxing the LES valve, so they may contribute to symptoms of acid reflux. Speak to your doctor about potential concerns you might have with these medications.

Herbal Remedies

While not considered to be medications per se, some herbs have properties that might be helpful for digestive disorders, such as indigestion, ulcers, or acid reflux. However, there is little information using reliable evidence-based studies on products that are specific for acid reflux disease. Some herbs may not be helpful and should be avoided if you have symptoms of acid reflux. It is not advisable for pregnant women to use any of these preparations without the advice of her physician.

Potentially Helpful Herbal Treatments

People with digestive disorders often have more than one problem, such as hyperacidity, ulcers, mucus membrane irritation, and so on. The following herbs have several healing properties.

Herb	Location of Ailment	Properties
Cat's Claw	Digestive system Peptic ulcers	Anti-inflammatory
Camomile	Digestive system Indigestion Colic Gastritis Peptic ulcers	Anti-inflammatory Antispasmotic Anti-anxiety
Dandelion Root	Digestive system Indigestion Dyspepsia	Digestive bitter
Devil's Claw	Digestive system Dyspepsia	Digestive bitter
Ginger	Digestive system Dyspepsia	Digestive aid
Goldenseal	Digestive system Mucus membranes	Astringent action Anti-inflammatory Anti-infective
Lemon Balm	Digestive system Abdominal bloating	Antispasmodic
Licorice	Digestive system Peptic and duodenal Ulcers Gastritis	Protects lining of gastrointestinal tract and mucus-secreting cells
Meadowsweet	Digestive system Hyperacidity Indigestion Peptic ulcer disease	Anti-inflammatory Soothing, healing action on the gastrointestinal system
Peppermint	Digestive system Dyspepsia Gastritis	Carminative Antispasmodic
Slippery Elm	Digestive system Peptic ulcer disease Gastritis	Anti-inflammatory Protects lining of mucus membranes
Thyme	Digestive system Dyspepsia	Antispasmotic

Herbs That Might Not Be Helpful

Be sure to avoid these herbal remedies if you are experiencing heartburn and other acid reflux symptoms.

Herb	Adverse Effects
Garlic	Heartburn, flatulence, gastrointestinal upset (if more than 4 cloves a day)
Ginger	Heartburn, digestive upset (rare)

CHAPTER 6

Surgical Intervention

Case History: Steve

Steve is a 58-year-old steelworker who has had problems with GERD for the past 20 years. He initially tried over-the-counter preparations, which provided some relief for a few years, then he used the higher-dose H2-RAs and PPI prescription medications. Over the past 5 years, he has been experiencing minimal relief from his symptoms of pain. He feels that it is time to explore surgical options, which he hopes will improve his quality of life.

Did You Know...

The decision to turn to a surgical solution for gastroesophageal reflux disease should not be a first choice. If you are considering surgery, explore the surgical options and find out who has true expertise in this area of surgery.

Surgery should never be viewed as a first-line therapy for the treatment of acid reflux disease. Rigorously approach medical and lifestyle management before resorting to surgical intervention. In most cases, PPIs provide excellent control for the majority of patients. However, there are a small number of patients who do not respond to standard therapy for reasons not yet understood. They might feel that surgery is the answer to their compromised quality of life.

There are a number of standard procedures that might be undertaken by surgeons, using either an open abdominal or thoracic approach. More recent options include the use of minimally invasive laparoscopic surgery.

When undertaken on carefully selected patients, surgery can have a very positive influence on quality of life. Conversely, if patients who are not the best candidates use it, the quality of life issues might not be improved.

Primary Indications for Surgery

- Defective LES
- Inadequate esophageal clearance of reflux material into the stomach
- Abnormalities of the stomach that encourage reflux activity

People whose primary problem is a defective LES are the most likely to benefit from surgical intervention.

Associated Indications

- Risk factors for progressive or difficult-to-manage disease
- Advanced or complicated disease
- Reflux disease complicated by disease in the chest

Surgery may also be considered for patients who have responded well to acid suppression with PPI medications but do not wish to remain on long-term medications for a variety of reasons.

Surgical Procedures

When deciding on a surgical procedure, the surgeon will consider physical features and needs of the patient from an individual perspective, including the length of the esophagus and esophageal motility. Anti-reflux surgical procedures are categorized into those that create a complete fundoplication and those that create a partial fundoplication. How these surgical procedures prevent reflux is not completely understood.

Surgery does not necessarily provide permanent relief in all patients. Some may not respond to surgical intervention initially; in others, the fundoplication may "slip" or become loose, such that reflux and symptoms recur.

Complete Fundoplication

The Nissen procedure is an example of a complete fundoplication, which can be undertaken using an open abdominal approach, an approach through the chest, or a laparoscopic procedure. It involves pulling the upper part of the stomach upward toward the esophagus, turning it in a full circle wrap around the esophagus, and draping it around the lower esophagus in folds that are stitched or stapled.

Partial Fundoplication

The Belsey procedure is an example of a partial fundoplication, which is usually approached via the chest. It involves an incomplete wrap of the upper stomach around the esophagus.

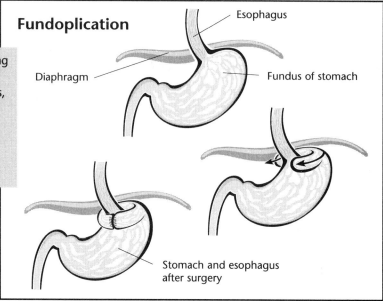

Fundoplication

Esophagus

Diaphragm

Fundus of stomach

Stomach and esophagus after surgery

A fundoplication involves pulling the upper part of the stomach upward toward the esophagus, turning it in a full circle wrap around the esophagus and draping it around the lower esophagus in folds that are stitched or stapled.

The procedure is preferred for those who have problems with peristalsis (the gentle wavelike muscle action that moves food through the intestinal tract) and have a low risk of swallowing problems following surgery.

Research studies suggest that the Nissen procedure might prove more effective in controlling reflux than the Belsey repair; however, some researchers suggest that there may be more post-operative problems with the Nissen procedure.

The Toupet partial fundoplication may provide some advantages over the Belsey approach. The Toupet procedure works well using a laparoscopic approach.

Surgical Complications

There are surgical complications that can occur. These are not always trivial.

- Gastroparesis (paralysis of the stomach) as a result of injury to the vagus nerve.
- Dysphagia (problems swallowing) could be a short-term problem as a result of tissue swelling after surgery, or it might be a long-term problem as a result of changes in esophageal motility that have occurred as a result of surgery.
- Recurrent problems with reflux.
- Inability to vomit.
- Gas bloat syndrome where patients feel bloated and unable to belch to relieve gas tension within the stomach.

Did You Know...

If a laparoscopic procedure is preferred to open surgery, carefully choose a center and a surgeon with significant expertise. The positive research findings using this procedure have been done in centers of excellence throughout North America. Small centers with minimal surgical expertise cannot be presumed to have the same success rates as the large academic and research facilities.

CHAPTER 7

Lifestyle Modifications

Case History: Ellen

Ellen has trouble managing her weight, which her doctor explains is a factor in her increasingly severe acid reflux symptoms. Her body mass index (BMI) of 44 is classified as Obesity, class III, on standard medical charts. Her waist circumference is 50 inches (125 cm), indicating central obesity. She is at risk of serious health problems that might occur due to her weight and waist circumference.

Ellen has tried many reducing regimens over the past 8 years; she loses some weight, but then gains it all back, along with some extra pounds. She is always on the lookout for a new diet regimen that might be "the answer" to her problem. At the same time, Ellen is also getting discouraged with continuing to try further weight reduction programs. She is feeling like something of a failure as a dieter.

Ellen is a working mom with three children between the ages of 4 and 8. She believes that she has no time or energy for physical activity. She feels too stressed and exhausted to plan for any changes right now . . .

(continued, page 60)

While there has been little research to determine if lifestyle modification is an effective treatment of chronic heartburn and acid reflux disease, it makes sense to consider key factors that can influence how the body functions when managing any health problem and to work at maximizing beneficial behaviors. Promoting good health involves evaluating your lifestyle and searching for behaviors or practices that might need to be adjusted to increase the chances of improving your overall sense of well-being. However, making lifestyle changes is not necessarily easy; if it were, we would all have made changes to our behavior long ago.

Start by considering what factors play a role in a healthy lifestyle. The primary lifestyle factors within our control are stress, exercise, and diet. Life in North American society can be challenging. The lifestyle we have grown accustomed to can make us particularly vulnerable to experiencing stress.

Did You Know...

Acid reflux is a disorder associated with increased symptoms in the presence of stressors, so an awareness of what causes stress and how to gain control over unhealthy aspects of stress is important in managing this condition.

Regular physical activity can act to reduce stress, improve muscle tone, and manage weight. Increasing body weight above recommended standards has been on the rise in Western societies, occurring at younger age ranges than in the past. Weight problems are rapidly becoming a major public health problem. Regular exercise and a healthy diet are the primary means of achieving and maintaining a healthy weight — and reducing the risk of acid reflux disease.

Lifestyle Health Factors

Regardless of what disease is being managed, it's important to consider your health with regard to key factors, such as:

- Stress
- Physical activity
- Eating habits
- Social interaction

Small Lifestyle Changes for Relief from Symptoms

In addition to modifying your lifestyle to reduce stress, increase physical activity, and manage your weight, these associated smaller changes may be helpful for managing GERD:

- Raise the head of the bed by about 6 inches (15 cm) using blocks, or raise the mattress or pillows using a special wedge, to enable gravity to control acid reflux.
- Avoid lying down for 3 hours after a meal.
- Discontinue smoking, because it acts to relax the LES, thereby increasing the risk of problems with acid reflux.
- Monitor the effect of alcohol use because it also acts to relax the LES.
- Wear loose-fitting clothes, especially around the abdominal area.
- Eat more slowly because rapid intake of food has been found to increase acid reflux symptoms.
- Avoid snacks between dinner and bedtime.
- Try to relax at mealtime because stress and anxiety can aggravate symptoms.

Stress Management

When we talk about stress, we often refer to a sense of tension or frustration that might occur throughout the day, linked to personal relationships that are not working out or personal goals that might not be achieved. For example, getting caught in traffic and being at risk of missing an important meeting might cause a sense of incredible frustration and anger, accompanied by anxiety and fear of what might happen as a result of not meeting our obligations to colleagues or clients. We may find meeting our obligations to our family equally stressful.

While some stress in our lives is normal and perhaps even healthy, chronic stress can lead to illnesses that can be life threatening for some. Normally, regulation of the stress response is tightly controlled by the body — it turns on when needed and then shuts down when not required. Problems arise for some people when the body is unable to regulate the stress response.

Stress Response

To preserve life, the human body is designed to flee quickly from a threatening situation to a place of safety or to stand and fight for survival, responses that were very useful to our ancestors when they encountered animals capable of destroying them and that remain useful today for anyone threatened with physical danger. This response to stress is commonly referred to as the "fight-or-flight" response. Within the brain, a signal is sent out to transport stress hormones throughout the body to prepare for the response to danger. The heart rate increases and breathing becomes more rapid. Mental focus and muscle strength increases, providing physical energy and strength.

Regulation of the stress hormones is a result of the action of three glands within the body: the hypothalamus, the pituitary gland, and the adrenal glands. Each gland produces hormones associated with the stress response. When we talk about the stress response within the body, we are referring to these three glands and the hormones they produce. The short form of describing the stress response is to call it the HPA axis — as in the hypothalamic, pituitary, adrenal axis.

Chronic Stress

While we continue to have the ability to mount this stress response to potential threats or irritants within our environment, the threat in our lives now tends to be more psychological than physical, based on our perception of stressors. Psychological stressors such as anxiety and constant worry about relationships, performance, and daily irritants can stimulate the response of stress hormones on a continuous basis within the body. As a result, unregulated stress hormones are often constantly present in our bodies, without being "turned off." This unregulated presence of stress hormones can influence the development of several chronic diseases, such as obesity, cardiovascular disease, depression, and certain cancers, as well as a variety of chronic inflammatory diseases.

Stress-Reducing Questions

Ask yourself the following questions as a way of taking stock of your stress. Your answers may lead to significant stress reduction.

Case History: Ellen

In addition to her problems at home, Ellen is angry about what she feels is an unfair division of the workload between herself and a colleague. She wants to speak to her boss but fears that if she speaks to him, the situation may worsen.

Ellen begins to feel drained. In response, she resorts to favorite foods to soothe her feelings. She chooses salted nuts and potato chips, which initially mask her anger. The food makes her feel a little better, but within a short time, she feels heartburn and acid reflux in her throat. In frustration, Ellen reaches for ice cream, which has often been a soother for her heartburn. In fact, it makes the situation worse. She has now consumed almost a thousand calories, which will interfere with her goal of losing weight. She needs antacids and some of her prescribed medications to treat the reflux symptoms immediately. The pain of ongoing heartburn is severe. She has no energy left to prepare dinner for the family. She can forget her earlier resolution to get some exercise. She is too exhausted.

This type of stress is not short term. Ellen is likely experiencing a chronic stress response, particularly since we know that she is also being challenged with long-term problems with significant obesity, a signal that unregulated stress hormones are likely a regular part of her life . . .

(continued, page 63)

- Is your view of the potential stressors in life accurate or might evaluating and perhaps changing your perspective be helpful?
- Could you make changes in your behavior that might help decrease stress in your life?
- Have you thought about learning to control your response to potential stressors by putting your body into a relaxed state?
- Have you thought about using physical activity to reduce your response to stress?

Physical Activity

Physical activity can be effective for reducing stress, enabling you to deal with emotional challenges, and controlling symptoms of chronic diseases, such as heartburn and acid reflux disease.

Physical activity can be defined as any body movement resulting from muscle contractions that increase the use of energy by the body. Within the body, food energy and physical activity are tightly linked. The three primary nutrients that provide energy to the body — carbohydrates, proteins, and fats — all facilitate physical movement, while at the same time physical activity regulates the use of these primary fuels.

Did You Know...

People who regularly engage in physical activity have been found to have a longer life span compared to those who are not active.

Q: How can you tell if you are physically fit?

A: People who are physically fit are described as having strong muscles, flexible joints, and a body that has not accumulated excessive fat. Those who are physically fit have the ability to engage in physical activity and still have reserve energy.

However, we live in a world that promotes physical inactivity. We are surrounded by labor-saving devices that require the use of minimal physical effort. As life becomes easier and less challenging physically, our level of fitness starts to decline and a host of chronic illnesses associated with lifestyle choices start to increase, chronic heartburn and acid reflux being prime examples. Research in the United States and Canada indicates that more than 60% of the population is not appropriately physically active.

Benefits of Regular Physical Activity

The Health Canada Physical Activity Guide lists the benefits of regular exercise:

- It feels good.
- It improves fitness.
- It provides a way to burn calories.
- It provides a way to regulate body weight.
- It improves overall body functioning — for example, digestive function.
- It enables stronger muscles and bones.
- It decreases the risk for chronic diseases.
- It is a de-stressor.

First Steps to Physical Fitness

Health Canada's Physical Activity Guide and the United States Department of Agriculture (USDA) MyPyramid activity guidelines recommend changing your lifestyle by taking the following first steps:

- Walk whenever possible.
- Use the stairs instead of the elevator.
- Walk short distances where in the past you might have driven or taken the transit system.
- Begin a formal walking program, starting with 10–15 minutes a day.
- Try using a pedometer to measure your progress each day.
- Reduce long periods of inactivity at work or at home.
- When you have a break from work, take a walk outside.
- Consider cycling or swimming.
- Consider joining an exercise class.

Exercise Programs

Exercise can be defined as repetitive body movements that act to promote physical fitness. Starting an exercise program does not have to be time-consuming or a complex addition to what is happening right now in your life. It's important to do exercise that you enjoy — also choose more than one activity, to enable your body to work out more than one muscle group. Variety is important in planning exercises for your regular routine.

Kinds of Physical Activity

Health Canada Physical Activity Guidelines and the United States Department of Agriculture (USDA) MyPyramid activity guidelines recommend including a variety of exercises in your routine several times each week. Alternate among the three basic kinds of physical activity.

Kinds of Exercise

Exercise	Duration	Example
Endurance exercise	4–7 days per week	Continuous walking, biking, swimming
Flexibility exercise	4–7 days per week	Gentle reaching, bending, stretching
Strength exercise	2–4 days per week	Resistance weightlifting, sit-ups, curls

Energy Burned

Activity	Kilocalories burned per hour
Bicycle riding, 6 miles (10 km) an hour	240
Jogging, 5 miles (8 km) an hour	740
Cross-country skiing	700
Swimming	275–500
Walking, 2 miles (3 km) an hour	240
Walking, 3 miles (5 km) an hour	320

Case History: Ellen

The last time Ellen met with her doctor, she indicated that she had no time for planned physical activity. Besides, she felt that running around after the needs of her children was enough of a workout.

Her doctor explained that this kind of physical activity is actually a form of stress that will gradually leave her feeling exhausted rather than refreshed and energized, the way that planned physical activity does. He advises her to make time for planned activities so she can "nurture" herself.

This is not selfish time; it's an opportunity to look after her needs, to regenerate energy, and to see to her personal requirements. Women have been socialized to look after others first, and often run out of time when it comes to dealing with their own needs. Physical activity can help her to improve self-esteem and mood disorders, manage her stress and weight — and control her acid reflux disease.

Weight Management

Problems with overweight and obesity are becoming epidemic in Western nations and affect people of all ages. The inability to maintain a healthy weight is resulting in associated major health problems, which include stress and fatigue, insulin resistance, type 2 diabetes, cardiovascular disease, hypertension, and osteoarthritis, to name a few conditions. Proper weight management has also been identified as a significant problem in people who are troubled by chronic heartburn and acid reflux. There are suggestions in the research literature that reducing body weight can improve some symptoms.

Overweight and obesity are challenging problems. Attempts at long-term weight loss are frequently disappointing for a number of reasons. Weight reduction is not as easy as just saying, use "will power" and reduce your dietary intake. Sometimes people eat food for reasons that have nothing to do with hunger. Inadequate physical activity, along with life stressors, can often interfere with attempts at losing weight or maintaining a healthy weight.

Q: What is a healthy body weight?

A: Determining your healthy body weight depends upon many factors, including your build, age, and diet. Healthy weight is:
- A weight that is appropriate for physical build or height
- A weight that is realistic for age
- A weight that is acceptable, based on inherited body shape and size
- A weight that can be achieved without constant dieting, but is based on healthy eating habits and regular physical activity

Measuring Overweight and Obesity

There are several accepted methods of measuring healthy weight and overweight, including the body mass index and the central obesity scales.

Body Mass Index (BMI)

One of the measures to classify overweight and obesity is called the body mass index (BMI). The BMI is an approximation of body fat for healthy individuals. It is calculated using the following formula:

> **Weight (kg)/Height (m^2) = BMI**
> *or*
> **Weight (lb) x 703/Height (in^2) = BMI**

Measuring weight in kilograms and height in meters
• Weight (lbs) divided by 2.2 = weight in kg
• Height (inches) multiplied by 2.5 = height in cm
• 100 centimeters = 1 meter

Let's use an example: Ellen's progressive problems with obesity have resulted in her developing problems with chronic heartburn and acid reflux, which are becoming worse. She has gained about 100 lbs (45.5 kg) over 8 years. She is about 5 feet, 4 inches tall (64 inches), or 160 cm (1.6 m). Her current weight is about 250 lbs or 113.6 kg. Her waist circumference is 50 inches, or about 125 cm.

BMI Calculation: Height = 1.6 m   Weight= 113.6 kg
$$113.6/(1.6)^2 = 113.6/2.56 = 44 \text{ BMI}$$

For those people with a computer Internet link, an easy way to determine BMI is to search for a BMI calculator site and key in your height and weight data to determine your BMI quickly.

Q: Is BMI an ideal measure for the classification of weight?

A: No. For some people, a BMI measure will not accurately reflect a healthy weight. This is because BMI provides an approximate estimate of body fat in healthy people, but not a true measure. BMI measures do not reflect healthy weights in the following situations:
- Women who are pregnant
- People with minimal muscle mass, such as the frail elderly
- Athletes with a large proportion of muscle mass
- Those who are dehydrated

Classification of Overweight and Obesity

To determine if your BMI is healthy, most health-care professionals and the World Health Organization use the following scales:

Classification	BMI
Underweight	<18.5
Normal	18.5–24.9
Overweight	25.0–29.9
Obesity, class I	30.0–34.9
Obesity, class II	35.0–39.9
Obesity, class III	40

Central Obesity

Central obesity measures are particularly important because they give an indication of how and where the body is storing adipose tissue. Measures of central obesity, in conjunction with BMI, provide a clear idea of the risk of chronic disease states linked to obesity. It is a good idea to evaluate the distribution of body fat and abdominal fat by measuring waist circumference. Just take a tape measure and do a waist measurement.

Central obesity–related health problems are a risk if the circumference is:

- Greater than 35 inches (88 cm) for women
- Greater than 40 inches (102 cm) for men

Improving Nutrition

If you have put on weight, achieving and maintaining a healthy weight is not an easy task. You need to manage stress, increase regular physical activity, and improve your nutrition. By improving your daily nutrition, you can reduce the risk of developing chronic heartburn and acid reflux disease. Avoiding foods that aggravate symptoms of acid reflux and selecting foods that prevent symptoms is also essential in a successful treatment plan for this disease. Good nutrition and diet guidelines are the subject of our next chapter.

Did You Know...

Overweight and obesity have been identified as risk factors for the development and aggravation of gastroesophageal reflux. Research studies suggest body weight has a direct influence on the function of the LES valve; in fact, when weight loss regimens are successful, symptoms of GERD have been found to decrease in some studies.

Good Nutrition and Diet Plans

CHAPTER 8

Food Basics

Case History: Jane

Jane is a 36-year-old nurse who works on a medical ward at the local hospital. She has had problems with heartburn for the past 6 years, requiring the regular use of prescription medications. In addition to being a full-time nurse, she is married with 3 children. She does not take time to plan her meals well. Meals are often missed during the day, while snacks of cookies, potato chips, or chocolate bars have become common over the past year.

When there is chance to sit down to a meal, Jane tends to grab anything that is convenient at the hospital, often reaching for a burger and fries with a can of pop. Her symptoms of heartburn have been increasing in severity over the past 9 months, despite using prescribed medications, and her weight has been rising as well. Perhaps it's time for her to evaluate her diet and lifestyle.

Did You Know...

When evaluating the role of diet in managing chronic heartburn and acid reflux disease, we need to understand the role of macronutrients and micronutrients in good nutrition and the acidic properties of foods that often aggravate symptoms of reflux.

The body needs a regular supply of energy, or calories, to enable it to function. The food we eat provides that energy using three major nutrients, or macronutrients: carbohydrates, proteins, and fats. Macronutrients are found in varying proportions within food, and each macronutrient contributes to the overall calories contained within food. Food also contains micronutrients, chiefly minerals and vitamins, which enable the major metabolic reactions involving carbohydrates, proteins, and fats to go on within the body. Minerals and vitamins are the key to facilitating all of the major chemical reactions throughout the body.

A healthy diet consists of a balance of macronutrients and micronutrients. Healthy eating can assist in weight loss and management — and in controlling and perhaps preventing acid reflux disease. However, while some of these food properties help to heal acid reflux disease, others may aggravate symptoms, depending upon the kind and quantity consumed. Whether to follow the suggestions on controlling dietary irritants and modifying diet to maintain a healthy weight is an individual decision. We all experience heartburn and accompanying symptoms in our own way. It's important to know what brings on and what controls heartburn for you. Choose food that helps to prevent the pain of heartburn.

Q: **What should my energy or calorie intake be per day?**

A: Energy requirements depend upon several factors: your height, weight, and age, as well as your current weight in relation to normal or ideal body weight, and how much energy you burn during daily activities and physical exercise. The energy contained in food is measured in calories, usually expressed as kilocalories (kcalories). Not everyone will have the same energy requirements.

To determine your energy requirements, look to the national food guides developed in Canada and the United States — Canada's Food Guide to Healthy Eating and the United States Department of Agriculture (USDA) MyPyramid. These will help you to plan meals using a variety of foods that will provide adequate energy, as well as vitamins and minerals. At the MyPyramid website (www.mypyramid.gov), you can enter your current height, weight, and activity level into their food planner, which will then recommend what calorie intake would be potentially appropriate for you, along with information on how many choices should be taken from each food group. The American Dietetic Association and the Dietitians of Canada have data on healthy eating and evaluation of how to maximize nutritional health. See the Resources section of the book for these listings. You can also consult your doctor or a registered dietitian.

Macronutrients

Macronutrients comprise carbohydrates (including fiber), proteins, and fats. They are found at different levels in various foods.

Carbohydrates

Carbohydrates are the primary source of energy for the body and the preferred fuel for the brain and nervous system. When you hear the term "carbohydrates," think of plant-based products rich in fiber, starches, and simple sugars. There are two main groups of carbohydrates: simple and complex carbohydrates. There are two groups of fiber: insoluble and soluble sources. Each has different actions within the body.

Kinds of Carbohydrates
Simple carbohydrates
• Fruits
• Honey
• Refined sugars
• Candy
Complex carbohydrates
• Starch sources (such as legumes, lentils, grains, cereals)
• Fiber sources (such as wheat bran, oat bran, oatmeal, barley, seeds)

Kinds of Fiber

Insoluble fiber provides roughage that facilitates the movement of waste through the intestinal tract, thereby preventing constipation. Digestive enzymes do not break down insoluble fiber as it moves through the intestinal tract. Bacteria within the colon ferment the fiber and provide a source of short-chain fatty acids to the body.

Soluble fiber arises from sticky carbohydrate sources, such as oatmeal, oat bran, barley, bananas, and applesauce. It dissolves in water to form a gel. Soluble fiber is readily used within the small bowel. It has a primary role in removing cholesterol from the body via the excretion of bile acids in the stool.

Carbohydrate Digestion

Digestive enzymes within the saliva begin the process of breaking down dietary starches. When carbohydrates move into the stomach, the acidic environment turns off the process of starch digestion. Then as starches move out of the stomach, enzymes from the pancreas take over the job of further digestion in the small bowel. However, fiber and some resistant complex starches are digested lower down in the digestive system, in the large bowel (colon), where resident bacteria act on them, producing some energy, as well as a great deal of fermentation products that can result in intestinal gas formation.

As carbohydrates move along the digestive tract, their digestion and the speed at which they are absorbed are affected by the type of fiber. Soluble and insoluble fibers move along the digestive tract at different speeds and with different actions. Water is a crucial element when consuming fiber because it facilitates the bulking up of intestinal contents with fiber to enable it to move through the system more readily, resulting in greater regulation of bowel function and movements, preventing problems with constipation.

Q: Is carbohydrate important in acid reflux disease?

A: Some researchers suggest that one of the problems with the dietary habits of Western societies is that refined sugar-type carbohydrates are consumed to excess, while unrefined complex carbohydrates are taken less frequently. The consumption of highly refined carbohydrates might be associated with an increased occurrence of many digestive diseases, including acid reflux disease. Heavy starchy-type foods are not readily digested within the stomach and are often delayed in leaving the stomach. The delay in exiting from the stomach can contribute to a feeling of bloating and overall discomfort. Starches and sugars that are not well digested within the gastrointestinal tract tend to ferment within the large bowel, causing a reflex "feedback" reaction all the way back up to the LES valve, increasing problems with acid reflux.

Did You Know...

Some recent research studies suggest that dietary fiber, as a result of its property of moving waste through the digestive system, is an important component of a healthy eating plan for people with acid reflux disease, reducing the symptoms of bloating and abdominal discomfort following a meal as a result of disordered motility. Dietary fiber can be helpful in this situation, particularly if a mixture of insoluble and soluble fibers is consumed.

Dietary Fiber Guidelines

Fiber found in carbohydrates is important in regulating the movement of digestive waste through the digestive system. The natural bacteria that reside in the colon ferment fiber and form an energy source called short-chain fatty acids that the body uses. In addition, soluble fiber in foods has been found to assist in lowering cholesterol within the body through linking with bile acids.

Adequate fluid intake is crucial to enable the action of fibrous products in the diet. Eight to 10 glasses of water a day is recommended to maintain fluid balance and to enable fiber to be used adequately within the body.

When increasing the intake of dietary fiber, it's important to work up the quantity gradually so the digestive system can adapt to the volume of indigestible carbohydrate provided by fiber. Indigestible carbohydrate foods tend to be fermented in the lower bowel, which, in the short term, may be irritating and uncomfortable to those troubled with cramps and gas. Gradual introduction of a higher fiber intake will help the bowel progressively adapt.

Fiber Food Diary

Eating dietary fiber in recommended amounts each day promotes good health and improves the symptoms of acid

Recommended Dietary Intake

The U.S. National Academy of Sciences recommends the following daily intake of fiber for those between the ages of 19 and 50 years:

- About 25 g per day for women
- About 38 g per day for men

reflux disease. To help you meet your recommended daily dietary fiber intake level, try using this chart. Check off (✓) sources of dietary fiber that you have consumed. Were you able to include food sources of fiber at each meal and snack? If not, what are some ways that you might make changes in your eating pattern to incorporate fiber on a regular basis?

Meals	Food Groups				
	Grains, cereals, rice, pasta	Milk, milk products	Fruits	Vegetables	Meats, meat substitutes, legumes, beans, nuts
Breakfast					
Morning Snack					
Lunch					
Afternoon Snack					
Dinner					
Evening Snack					

Proteins

Proteins are a key nutrient found in all tissues within the body. Primary food sources of this nutrient are animal-based products, such as meats, eggs, legumes, lentils, and nuts and seeds, as well as dairy products. Unlike carbohydrates and fats, proteins are not a primary source of energy; instead, they play a key role in the building and repair of tissues, providing structure within the body and regulating chemical reactions and fluid balance. In addition, protein is closely linked to immune system function.

Protein Digestion

Consuming adequate dietary protein is crucial to maintaining overall health. The primary digestion of protein occurs in the stomach, where hydrochloric acid breaks down food sources of this nutrient before it progresses to the small bowel for further digestion by specialized pancreatic enzymes.

Fats

Dietary fats are energy dense, providing more kilocalories in a smaller volume than carbohydrates and proteins. Fats are just as important for the maintenance of health as the other two macronutrients. They also provide an important source of essential fatty acids and act as carriers of essential fat-soluble vitamins.

Q: Does protein have an impact on acid reflux disease?

A: Protein probably has an effect on acid reflux. If it is digested slowly, this leads to delayed emptying of the stomach and increased acid secretion. Protein, peptides, and peptones are potent stimuli for the secretion of stomach acid.

Fats are part of a family of lipids, which include triglycerides, phospholipids, and sterols, all of which have unique and important roles within the body. Triglycerides have the ability to be compactly stored within adipose tissue cells, where a ready source of energy is available to the body. Adipose tissue stores of fat also influence the secretion of significant hormones, as well as the production of enzymes that exert control over appetite and influence how the body uses energy. Phospholipids are important in the maintenance of cell membranes within the body, while sterols are essential for the body's survival.

Fats Digestion

The movement of fat through the digestive tract is relatively slow. Digestion of fats begins in the small intestine, not in the stomach. Unabsorbed fat, either as a result of excessive intake or impaired digestion, can cause loose stools (steatorrhea), with gastrointestinal symptoms of urgency and frequency of bowel movements.

Q: Is fat important in acid reflux disease?

A: Most people who experience significant symptoms of acid reflux disease say that heavy, greasy foods aggravate symptoms. Meals rich in fat content can remain in the stomach for hours, causing a sense of fullness and possibly interfering with lower esophageal sphincter valve function. Slower emptying of the stomach may be a factor in disordered motility. Problems with emptying the stomach contribute to inappropriate relaxation of the LES, enabling acid reflux to continue.

There is a recognized phenomenon called the ileal brake, which explains many of the symptoms that people experience. When undigested food reaches the small bowel from the stomach, a feedback mechanism occurs, whereby a signal is given to slow down the emptying of the stomach and to slow down the movement of food through the small bowel to facilitate digestion. At the same time, the stomach begins to slow down the process of emptying content into the small bowel. The result is an increase in reflux back into the esophagus.

The balance of macronutrients in a meal will strongly influence the movement of fat through the digestive tract. The emptying of the stomach after a meal can take anywhere from 2 to 6 hours. Fat tends to be the last macronutrient that leaves the stomach, so if the meal is rich in fat, movement will be slow compared to a meal that is low in fats and high in carbohydrates.

Dietary Fat Guidelines

The recommendations for total daily fat intake are expressed as a percentage of total energy or calorie intake. The U.S. National Academy of Sciences recommends the following levels:

- Age 1–3 years: 30%–40% of total energy intake
- Age 4–18 years: 25%–35% of total energy intake
- Age 19+ years: 20%–35% of total energy intake

For adults from age 19 and above, the recommendations for dietary fat are 20% to 35% of total energy intake. So if total energy intake is 2000 kilocalories, then the suggested daily intake of fat would be a range between 44 g and 78 g a day. If total energy intake is 1500 kilocalories, then the suggested range of intake would be between 33 g to 58 g a day.

Micronutrients

Micronutrients are essential to the normal functioning of the body. They are not produced within the body, but are available in the foods consumed in a healthy diet. Minerals and vitamins are the chief micronutrients found in our food. Many minerals are important for the maintenance of body structures, such as bones and tissue, and for enabling a host of metabolic reactions in the body. Vitamins are important as chemical factors that allow other nutrients to be digested, absorbed, and metabolized. Most chemical reactions involving the macronutrients require minerals or vitamins to facilitate the body's metabolic activity, which is not constant, but reacts to other activities, needs, and stressors.

Meal Size and Frequency

The size and frequency of meals seems to have an influence on the symptoms of acid reflux disease. Small meals that are balanced with respect to macronutrient composition and taken more frequently tend to be better tolerated than larger meals, which might not empty from the stomach in a predictable manner.

When eating large meals, the stomach is filled with food that may move into the small bowel very slowly. A stomach that remains full for hours may contribute to exerting pressure on the lower esophageal sphincter and causing a weakening of the LES muscle. The end result might be more problems with the backup of acid from the stomach into the esophagus, causing acid reflux and heartburn.

Healthy Diet Guidelines

The United States Department of Agriculture (USDA) and Health Canada publish healthy eating guidelines developed by nutrition experts, called MyPyramid and Canada's Food Guide to Healthy Eating (CFGHE), respectively. Use either of these guidelines as a framework for planning meals if you or a family member is experiencing acid reflux disease. A healthy diet is beneficial beyond the control of symptoms of chronic heartburn and acid reflux.

Food Groups

The importance of eating a variety of foods from each food group each day is advocated to promote health by both recognized food guides. You can use these food guides to ensure that meals are balanced and contain macronutrients from each food group.

Each food guide classifies macronutrient foods into groups that have similar nutrients per serving. For example, meats and alternatives are primary sources of protein and fat; breads and cereals are primary sources of carbohydrates and protein; and dairy products contain carbohydrates, protein, and often fat. Within the recognized guides, foods are categorized based on their composition: for example, Meat and Alternatives is the primary group for protein-rich foods,

Macronutrient Food Groups

Food Guide	Grain Products	Vegetables & Fruit	Milk Products	Meat & Alternatives
Carbohydrate	Carbohydrate	Carbohydrate	Carbohydrate	Carbohydrate
Fat			Fat	Fat
Protein	Protein		Protein	Protein

such as meats, fish, poultry, and eggs, but legumes and lentils also contain carbohydrates; the Milk Products group consists of protein foods from dairy sources; the Grain Products group consists of foods that are primarily complex carbohydrates with a small amount of protein, and so on.

Recommended Daily Intake of Macronutrients

Carbohydrates

Carbohydrate intake should be moderate, providing 25 to 35 g of dietary fiber a day. Primary food sources of fiber are whole-grain breads and cereals, vegetables, fruits, nuts, and seeds.

Proteins

Daily protein intake should be about 1 g of protein per 2.2 lbs of body weight, or at least 1 g protein per kg body weight. Key food sources of protein are meats, poultry, fish, eggs, and dairy products. The national food guides provide information on how to provide adequate daily protein by providing a variety of food from each food group.

Fats

Total dietary fat intake should be moderate, controlling the use and portion size of saturated animal fats, while substituting mono- and polyunsaturated fats.

Trans fatty acids from commercially prepared products, such as baked goods, certain peanut butter products, and convenient snack foods, should not be consumed on a regular basis. Reading product labels will identify those that contain trans fatty acids.

Providing omega-3 fatty acids in the diet is important. Primary food sources are salmon oil, smoked salmon, herring, shrimp, trout, halibut, tuna, crab, canola oil, ground flaxseeds, and walnuts.

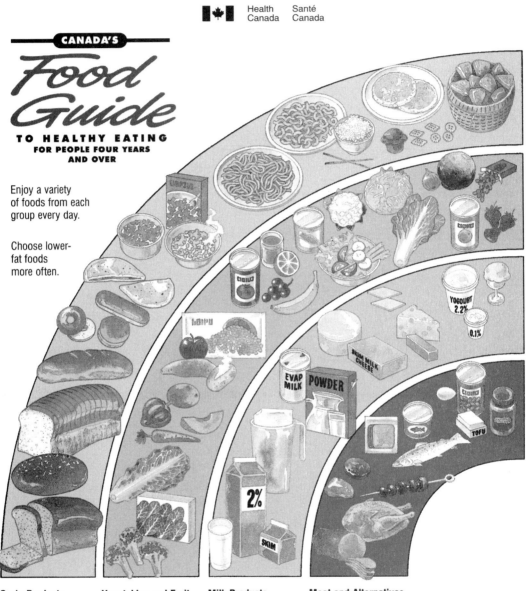

Health Canada Santé Canada

CANADA'S
Food Guide
TO HEALTHY EATING
FOR PEOPLE FOUR YEARS AND OVER

Enjoy a variety of foods from each group every day.

Choose lower-fat foods more often.

Grain Products
Choose whole grain and enriched products more often.

Vegetables and Fruit
Choose dark green and orange vegetables and orange fruit more often.

Milk Products
Choose lower-fat milk products more often.

Meat and Alternatives
Choose leaner meats, poultry and fish, as well as dried peas, beans and lentils more often.

Canada

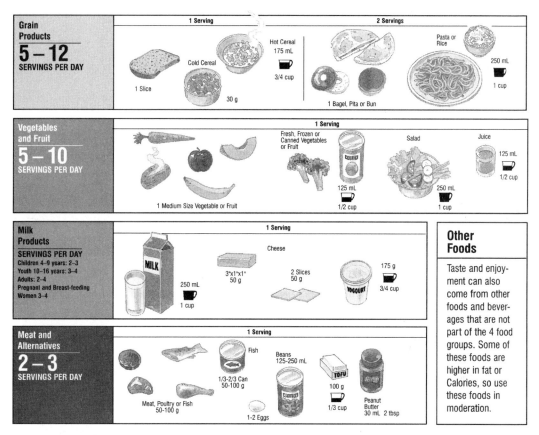

Grain Products

5 – 12 SERVINGS PER DAY

1 Serving
1 Slice
Cold Cereal 30 g
Hot Cereal 175 mL 3/4 cup

2 Servings
1 Bagel, Pita or Bun
Pasta or Rice 250 mL 1 cup

Vegetables and Fruit

5 – 10 SERVINGS PER DAY

1 Serving
1 Medium Size Vegetable or Fruit
Fresh, Frozen or Canned Vegetables or Fruit 125 mL 1/2 cup
Salad 250 mL 1 cup
Juice 125 mL 1/2 cup

Milk Products

SERVINGS PER DAY
Children 4–9 years: 2–3
Youth 10–16 years: 3–4
Adults: 2–4
Pregnant and Breast-feeding Women 3–4

1 Serving
MILK 250 mL 1 cup
Cheese 3"x1"x1" 50 g
2 Slices 50 g
Yogourt 175 g 3/4 cup

Other Foods

Taste and enjoyment can also come from other foods and beverages that are not part of the 4 food groups. Some of these foods are higher in fat or Calories, so use these foods in moderation.

Meat and Alternatives

2 – 3 SERVINGS PER DAY

1 Serving
Meat, Poultry or Fish 50-100 g
Fish 1/3-2/3 Can 50-100 g
1-2 Eggs
Beans 125-250 mL
Tofu 100 g
1/3 cup
Peanut Butter 30 mL 2 tbsp

Different People Need Different Amounts of Food

The amount of food you need every day from the 4 food groups and other foods depends on your age, body size, activity level, whether you are male or female and if you are pregnant or breast-feeding. That's why the Food Guide gives a lower and higher number of servings for each food group. For example, young children can choose the lower number of servings, while male teenagers can go to the higher number. Most other people can choose servings somewhere in between.

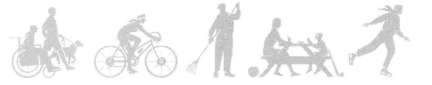

Consult *Canada's Physical Activity Guide to Healthy Active Living* to help you build physical activity into your daily life.

Enjoy eating well, being active and feeling good about yourself. That's VITALIT®

© Minister of Public Works and Government Services Canada, 1997
Cat. No. H39-252/1992E   ISBN 0-662-19648-1

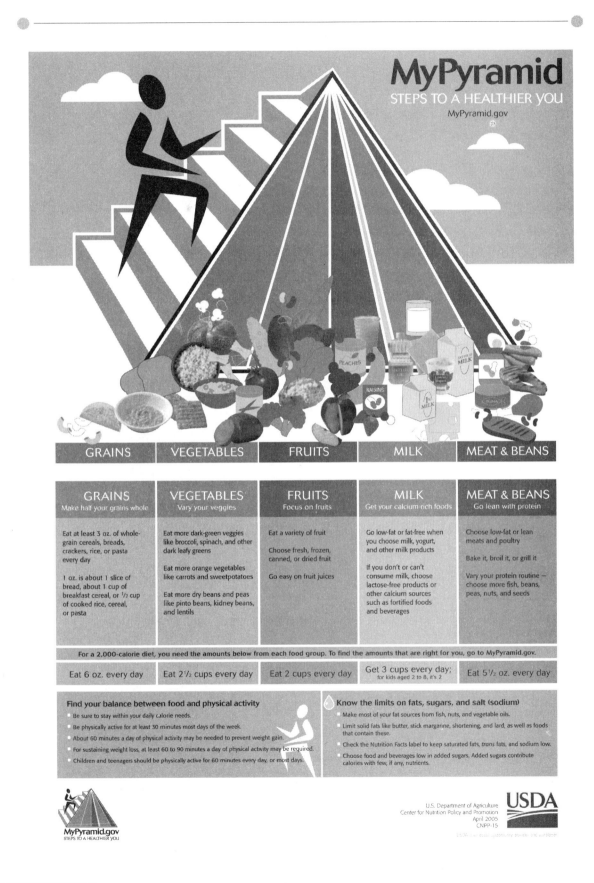

MyPyramid
STEPS TO A HEALTHIER YOU
MyPyramid.gov

GRAINS	VEGETABLES	FRUITS	MILK	MEAT & BEANS
GRAINS Make half your grains whole	**VEGETABLES** Vary your veggies	**FRUITS** Focus on fruits	**MILK** Get your calcium-rich foods	**MEAT & BEANS** Go lean with protein
Eat at least 3 oz. of whole-grain cereals, breads, crackers, rice, or pasta every day 1 oz. is about 1 slice of bread, about 1 cup of breakfast cereal, or ½ cup of cooked rice, cereal, or pasta	Eat more dark-green veggies like broccoli, spinach, and other dark leafy greens Eat more orange vegetables like carrots and sweetpotatoes Eat more dry beans and peas like pinto beans, kidney beans, and lentils	Eat a variety of fruit Choose fresh, frozen, canned, or dried fruit Go easy on fruit juices	Go low-fat or fat-free when you choose milk, yogurt, and other milk products If you don't or can't consume milk, choose lactose-free products or other calcium sources such as fortified foods and beverages	Choose low-fat or lean meats and poultry Bake it, broil it, or grill it Vary your protein routine — choose more fish, beans, peas, nuts, and seeds

For a 2,000-calorie diet, you need the amounts below from each food group. To find the amounts that are right for you, go to MyPyramid.gov.

| Eat 6 oz. every day | Eat 2½ cups every day | Eat 2 cups every day | Get 3 cups every day; for kids aged 2 to 8, it's 2 | Eat 5½ oz. every day |

Find your balance between food and physical activity
- Be sure to stay within your daily calorie needs.
- Be physically active for at least 30 minutes most days of the week.
- About 60 minutes a day of physical activity may be needed to prevent weight gain.
- For sustaining weight loss, at least 60 to 90 minutes a day of physical activity may be required.
- Children and teenagers should be physically active for 60 minutes every day, or most days.

Know the limits on fats, sugars, and salt (sodium)
- Make most of your fat sources from fish, nuts, and vegetable oils.
- Limit solid fats like butter, stick margarine, shortening, and lard, as well as foods that contain these.
- Check the Nutrition Facts label to keep saturated fats, trans fats, and sodium low.
- Choose food and beverages low in added sugars. Added sugars contribute calories with few, if any, nutrients.

MyPyramid.gov
STEPS TO A HEALTHIER YOU

U.S. Department of Agriculture
Center for Nutrition Policy and Promotion
April 2005
CNPP-15

USDA

Key Nutritional Recommendations to Promote Health

- Eat a variety of foods from each food group daily while staying within energy limits (caloric intake).
- Place emphasis on whole-grain cereals, breads, and grain products within the daily meal plan.
- Consume 25 to 38 g of dietary fiber daily.
- Eat adequate amounts of fruits and vegetables daily.
- Choose lean meats and lower-fat milk and dairy products.
- Choose fats wisely, limiting sources of saturated fats from animal-based products and tropical oils.
- Limit salt, alcohol, and caffeine use.
- Make food choices that will promote a healthy body weight.

Dietary Guidelines for Acid Reflux

When planning a diet regimen for people with acid reflux disease, these healthy eating guidelines provide the foundation for meal planning. However, the dietary management of each individual will vary to some degree because individuals do not all experience the disease in the same way, nor do they all tolerate the same foods.

Recommended Daily Servings

Canada's Food Guide to Healthy Eating Food groups (1800 kcalories per day)	Servings per day	USDA MyPyramid Food groups (1800 kcalories per day)	Servings per day
Grain Products	7–8	Breads, cereals, rice, pasta	6 oz-eq (175 g)
Vegetables and Fruit	7–8 (½ cup/ 125 mL portions)	Vegetables Fruit	2½ cups (625 mL) 1½ cups (375 mL)
Milk Products	7–8 (½ cup/ 125 mL portions)	Milk, yogurt, cheese	3 cups
Meat and Alternatives	6 oz-eq (175 g)	Meat, poultry, fish, eggs, dried beans, nuts	5 oz-eq (150 g)
Other Foods: Fats/Oils Sugars	Use in moderation (5–6 tsp/25–30 mL)	Fats, oils, sweets	Use sparingly

Q: How do I know how many servings of each food group should be eaten each day?

A: The food guides provide a range of serving sizes to accommodate the needs of different people, at different ages and at different stages in the life cycle. Here are two cases:

Tom is a physically active adolescent who is growing normally. The daily recommended food servings within each food group would be at the maximum suggested.

Food Groups	Canada's Food Guide	USDA MyPyramid Food Guide
for 3200 kcalories		
Grains, cereals	14–15	10 oz-eq (300 g)
Vegetables, fruit	12–14 (½ cup/ 125 mL portions)	4 cups (1 L) 2½ cups (625 mL)
Milk products	8 (½ cup/ 125 mL portions)	3 cups (750 mL)
Meat & alternatives	8 oz-eq (250 g)	7 oz-eq (200 g)
Other foods: fats/ oils, sweets	Moderate use (13–14 tsp/65–70 mL)	11 tsp (55 mL)

Tammy is a 55-year-old mother. She runs a household and works full-time in a stressful job. She is often too tired to exercise on a regular basis. The daily food servings would be somewhere in the middle range of suggested servings. When Tammy begins to increase physical activity, the servings taken each day can then be increased.

Food Groups	Canada's Food Guide	USDA MyPyramid Food Guide
for 1600 kcalories		
Grains, cereals	6	5 oz-eq (150 g)
Vegetables, fruit	6–7 (½ cup/ 125 mL portions)	2 cups (500 mL) 1½ cups (375 mL)
Milk products	6 (½ cup/ 125 mL portions)	3 cups (750 mL)
Meat & alternatives	5 oz-eq (150 g)	5 oz-eq (150 mL)
Other foods: fats/ oils, sweets	Moderate use (4–5 tsp/20–25 mL)	5 tsp (25 mL)

For all individuals with acid reflux:

- Eat a low-fat diet to prevent relaxation of the lower esophageal sphincter muscle and acid reflux from the stomach.
- Avoid foods that can act to relax the LES muscle:
  - High-fat foods, frying with fats and oils
  - Garlic, onions, radishes, peppers
  - Chocolate
  - Mint, peppermint
  - Alcohol
  - Coffee, tea, cola, and other caffeine products
  - Carbonated beverages, such as soda pop
- Avoid foods that can irritate the lining of the esophagus:
  - Citrus fruits and juices, such as lemon, lime, orange, and grapefruit
  - Tomato products, such as ketchup, chili, spaghetti sauce, pizza sauce
  - Vinegar-based products, such as mustard, salad dressings
  - Spicy foods
- Eat smaller meals, if necessary, more frequently throughout the day.
- Try to include protein foods with each meal and snack.
- Try to relax at mealtime: stress and anxiety can aggravate symptoms.
- Do not eat within 3 hours of going to bed.
- Do not lie down after eating because symptoms of acid reflux may be triggered, leading to related esophageal injury.

Did You Know...

There is not good evidence in the medical literature that a change in diet will heal damage caused by reflux disease.

For those with an additional weight problem:

A calorie-controlled diet might be indicated because pressure on the stomach will be increased, aggravating symptoms of acid reflux disease.

Three large meals taken over the day tends to contribute to increasing pressure within the stomach, so it's best to begin by eating six smaller meals over the day, to prevent a pressure buildup on the stomach secondary to the presence of food.

CHAPTER 9

Foods that Hurt, Foods that Heal

Case History: Jean

Jean is a 29-year-old public relations assistant in a large corporation. During the past year, she has been experiencing increasing problems with heartburn that are beginning to interfere with her quality of life. She has always enjoyed a breakfast that included fresh orange juice, toast, and peanut butter, along with a large, strong cup of coffee. Italian pasta with tomato sauce and cheese, along with a glass of wine, has been a favorite meal later in the day. Jean is dismayed that some of her favored foods have started to cause her significant heartburn, requiring medication and interfering with her productivity at work and her lifestyle.

Did You Know...

A "healthy diet" that makes your symptoms worse is not a healthy diet for you! Consult your doctor if diet does not help.

Not all foods, regardless of their nutritional values, can be comfortably consumed if you have chronic heartburn and acid reflux. Some foods can play a role in decreasing the muscle tone of the lower esophageal sphincter, while others might be direct irritants to esophageal tissue. These foods are not well tolerated. However, other foods are tolerated and still others are soothing, perhaps healing.

The foods identified here are the most common ones that predictably cause pain for the majority of people. However, each person might have some differences in foods that offend and those that are tolerated. Use the general information provided to maintain control over the pain of heartburn and acid reflux. The severity of the symptoms of gastroesophageal reflux disease, the presence of esophageal erosions, and differences in the speed at which food moves out of the stomach and through the digestive system might contribute in different ways to how people experience and tolerate different foods.

As acid reflux disease symptoms come under control, foods that were initially not tolerated may become less of a problem for some people. You may find greater freedom with tolerated foods.

Painful Foods

Acidic foods and drinks, as well as foods high in fats, are not well tolerated if you have acid reflux disease.

- Citrus juices and products
- Tomato products
- High-fat foods
- Caffeine (foods and beverages)
- Wines (white wines are sometimes more acidic than red wines)
- Alcoholic spirits
- Vinegar-based products
- Mint (all types)
- Chocolate
- Onions and garlic

Adverse Food Reactions

Food choices have been linked to some of the symptoms of acid reflux disease and have been found to be closely associated with transient relaxations of the lower esophageal sphincter muscle.

A general understanding of how the digestive system works in relation to the food going through this system is helpful when considering some of the symptoms of acid reflux disease that might relate to food choices.

Eating these foods can cause a number of physical reactions that compound the symptoms of acid reflux disease:

- Cause symptoms similar to reflux. Citrus fruits and drinks, carbonated drinks, spicy foods, and alcohol irritate the esophagus. Symptoms may occur during swallowing or after eating because the refluxed material acts as an irritant. These foods do not necessarily increase reflux.
- Cause reflux by affecting the LES muscle. Consuming chocolate and mint may lead to this reaction.

Did You Know...

Food diaries might be helpful in identifying which foods are difficult to tolerate when on and off medications for acid reflux disease.

- Cause reflux by stimulating increased secretion of acid and pepsin.
- Cause reflux by delaying the emptying of the stomach. This is most common when these foods are eaten just before lying down at nighttime or for a nap, resulting in an increase in the transient lower esophageal sphincter reactions. The result is increased problems with discomfort and bloating around the abdominal area.
- Cause reflux by inhibiting the reflux action of emptying the stomach. Because high-fat foods are slow to digest, they may be left over from a previous meal.
- Cause increased weight. These foods may lead to weight gain, placing mechanical strain on the anti-reflux barrier and an increasing risk of hiatus hernia.
- Cause increased acid secretion by the stomach. High-caloric load foods will increase the risk of acid reflux, particularly following meals.

Tolerated Foods

Some of the foods from the painful list might be tolerated some of the time:

- Sweet onions
- Regular tea — although it is a source of caffeine, tea is often tolerated
- Some alcohols, such as spirits
- Decaffeinated beverages

Comfortable Foods

- Lower-fat milk products: milk, yogurt, lower-fat cheeses
- Meat and substitutes: meats, poultry, and fish that are not pan-fried or deep-fried; legumes and lentils that are digestible
- Most fruits, particularly those that are canned
- Vegetables that are not deep-fried or acidic
- Breads and cereals that are not rich and greasy
- Herbal teas, such as mango, raspberry, and ginger

Food Tolerance Guide

Food Groups	Usually Tolerated	Not Well Tolerated
Cereals, grains, and breads	Breads, cereals, grains that are not rich in fat content; dry crackers, low-fat muffins; rice, pastas	Greasy, high-fat products, such as croissants, tea biscuits, pastries, pies, doughnuts, sweet rolls; pastas with rich, creamy sauces
Milk and milk products	Fat-free milk and low-fat yogurt, smoothies, cheese, cottage cheese, sour cream	Heavy cream, cream cheese, whole milk, milkshakes
Meat and alternatives	Lean meats, poultry, fish, eggs, low-fat cheese; legumes and all types of peas, lentils, and beans; soy products, tofu	Fried meats, poultry, eggs, sausage, bacon
Vegetables	Fresh, frozen, or canned vegetables prepared by steaming or boiling; peas, carrots, green beans, mushrooms, squash, zucchini, eggplant, spinach, salad greens; soups made from vegetables	Fried vegetables, tomatoes, tomato products, onions, vegetable juices; gaseous vegetables might be a temporary problem: cabbage, broccoli, cauliflower, Brussels sprouts, turnip; tomato and cream-type soups; french fries, potato chips
Fruits	Fresh, frozen, or canned fruits; non-acidic juices, such as mango, peach, pear, or berry varieties	Citrus juices, oranges, lemons, grapefruit, some apple juices
Desserts	Fruit sources tolerated, gelatins, fruit ices, sherbets, sorbet, low-fat puddings, custard; low-fat cakes, such as angel food; low-fat cookies	Chocolate desserts, whole-milk puddings, ice cream; rich cakes and cookies high in fat content
Sweets	Sugar, honey, maple syrup, hard candies	Chocolate
Snacks	Low-fat crackers; pretzels if tolerated	Nuts, potato chips
Fats and oils	Low-fat dressings and mayonnaise; small amounts of butter or margarine; vegetable oils	Gravy, meat drippings, bacon, generous amounts of butter, margarine, oils
Beverages	Herbal fruit teas	Carbonated beverages, coffee, mint teas, most alcoholic beverages
Miscellaneous	Salt, pepper, herbs as tolerated: sage, basil, oregano, tarragon, rosemary, etc.	Chili, strong spices, jalapeño peppers, vinegar products, mustards

Adapted by permission from the *Manual of Clinical Dietetics*, Chicago Dietetic Association, the South Suburban Dietetic Association, and the Dietitians of Canada. Chicago, IL: American Dietetic Association, 2000.

Food Diary

It's a good idea to keep a food diary when you are learning to recognize symptoms related to acid reflux. Some people tolerate foods that others cannot manage. A food diary can be helpful to identify foods that tend to trigger symptoms of acid reflux, so that meals can be planned to avoid those that irritate and include those that work well.

It's also important to note that sometimes you may find that foods that have given you a problem in the past might be tolerated when prescribed medication for acid reflux is being taken. The table below provides an example of how you might document the foods that are particularly upsetting.

Sample Food Tolerance Diary

Breakfast	Might Not Be Tolerated	Lunch	Might Not Be Tolerated	Dinner	Might Not Be Tolerated
Apple juice	✓	Vegetable soup		Grilled fish	
Egg		Turkey slices		Potatoes	
Bacon	✓	Cheese	✓	Peas	
High-fiber toast		Mustard	✓	Steamed carrots	
Peanut butter	✓	High-fiber bread		Plain bagel	✓
Coffee	✓	Spinach salad		Cherries	
		Onion, peppers	✓		
		Zucchini			
		Balsamic vinaigrette	✓		
		Olive oil			
		Lean roast beef sandwich (½) with tomato, onion and mustard	✓		
Snack		**Snack**		**Snack**	
Blueberry muffin	✓	Mango juice		Potato chips	✓
				Cola beverage	✓
				Canned fruit	

Food Tolerance Diary

Customize this diary to identify specific foods that may cause you problems. Make photocopies as needed.

Breakfast	Might Not Be Tolerated	Lunch	Might Not Be Tolerated	Dinner	Might Not Be Tolerated
Snack		Snack		Snack	

Food Tolerance Guide

Meal	Problem	Substitute
Breakfast		
Apple juice	Might be acidic	Try mango, peach, or pear nectar
Bacon	Might be too greasy and high in fat	Try low-fat yogurt
Peanut butter	Might be too high in fat	Try low-fat cheese
Coffee	Might be acidic	Try herbal fruit teas
Morning Snack		
Blueberry muffin	Might be too high in fat	Try a low-fat muffin or low-fat crackers and hummus (chickpea spread)
Lunch		
Cheese	Might be too high in fat	Try low-fat cheeses, flaked tuna, or lean sliced meats
Mustard	Too acidic	Try a small amount of mild low-fat dressing
Balsamic vinegar	Too acidic	Try a small amount of mild non-fat or low-fat dressing OR some extra-virgin olive oil
Onion, tomato, mustard	Might be too acidic and irritate the esophagus	Try lettuce in a sandwich with a small amount of margarine or low-fat mayonnaise (not one that contains vinegar)
Afternoon Snack		
Plain bagel	Might be difficult to digest	Try whole-grain bread
Dinner		
Plain bagel	Might be difficult to digest	Try whole-grain bread
Breaded chicken	Might be too high in fat and difficult to digest	Try baked or broiled chicken — remove the skin
French fries	Might be too high in fat and difficult to digest	Try baked or boiled potatoes or sweet potatoes
Grilled zucchini	Might be too greasy	Try steamed or baked zucchini, green peas, corn or string beans
Evening Snack		
Potato chips	Might be too greasy	Try baked chips or baked corn chips
Cola beverage	Difficult to digest	Try non-carbonated fruit drinks or juices that are tolerated

Food Substitution

For foods not tolerated with acid reflux, consider substitutes. To ensure that nutritional adequacy is being provided in meals each day, the dietary guidelines need to form the framework of meal planning, with appropriate substitutions for those foods that are not tolerated.

- If fried eggs or omelets are not tolerated, try boiled eggs, or perhaps an omelet prepared from egg whites, cooked in a nonstick pan that has been sprayed with a low-fat oil product.
- Instead of adding regular cheese, a low-fat product might be used.
- Vegetables such as mushrooms, cut-up green beans, spinach, water chestnuts, and other vegetables that are tolerated can also be added to an omelet.
- If a bagel and margarine or cream cheese is difficult to digest, try a slice of whole-grain toast with jelly or honey on top.

Note: Don't substitute with dips that may worsen reflux — such as salsa, cheese, and so on.

CHAPTER 10

Dietary Steps for Managing Chronic Heartburn

Case History: John

John is a 35-year-old teacher who has experienced intermittent problems with heartburn and acid reflux for about 7 years. During the past 6 months, he has needed to use over-the-counter medications to control symptoms of heartburn on a daily basis. Three weeks ago, his family doctor prescribed proton pump inhibitors to control the continuous pain that John has been experiencing.

The doctor also reminded John that it was time to review his usual eating patterns, as well as lifestyle activities that might be contributing to the progression of his symptoms. The doctor provided John with more diet information and started him on a restricted regimen at first, with food choices to be increased when the action of the medication begins to resolve his painful symptoms.

When dietitians plan meals for people with diseases that require some modification in food choices, they begin by considering which foods will likely be best tolerated. Even with severe pain, there are usually certain foods that will be tolerated. This is Step 1 in managing chronic heartburn and acid reflux with diet. Starting with a basic "foundation" diet regimen provides the opportunity to gain some confidence in managing your illness using foods that will not aggravate symptoms. As pain begins to come under control, more foods can be added to the foundation diet regimen. This is Step 2 in managing this condition. Most people find that they are able to tolerate larger portions at the three meals, taking smaller between-meal snacks and sometimes eliminating snacks. This is Step 3. Various menus and 7-day menu plans are recommended for each stage.

Step 1: Meal Plans When Pain Is Severe

To bring severe symptoms under control, start by being restrictive for the first couple of weeks and then gradually be less rigorous with restrictions. Food choices can then be expanded when heartburn and reflux come under control with the use of medications, such as the proton pump inhibitors. If there is a relapse of symptoms, greater restriction in food choices might be indicated until remission in symptoms comes under control once again.

Guidelines

- Start by avoiding foods you know from past experience trigger your symptoms of acid reflux, and those known to irritate esophageal tissue, such as acidic and spicy foods that will quickly bring on pain.
- Avoid foods that interfere with the lower esophageal sphincter (LES) muscle function, causing changes in the movement of food through the digestive system. These foods are often high in fat content, starchy, and low in fiber content, and they move out of the stomach more slowly, causing a significant feeling of bloating. Foods that may interfere with the LES muscle function are identified in Foods that Hurt, Foods that Heal, pages 84–91.
- When planning meals, it's a good idea to be guided by the severity of symptoms experienced, but it is also important to maintain a balanced diet regimen. So, don't limit your food choices excessively in the long term.
- Don't presume that a food that was once bothersome will remain that way forever — try it out.

Sample Meal Plan When Pain Is Severe

Let's start with the food groups. Using this basic diet plan, a menu for one day can be constructed that is low in fat and divided into six small meals. Six small meals means that portion sizes will be smaller.

> **Did You Know...**
>
> Do not confine yourself to a highly restricted diet based on fear of trying a greater variety of foods. Experiment with the addition of foods that have been initially avoided. The action of powerful medications to treat acid reflux disease will often provide opportunities to add variety to one's food choices.

Meals	Food Groups				
	Grains, cereals, rice, pasta, starches	Milk, milk products	Fruits	Vegetables	Meats, meat substitutes, legumes, beans, nuts
Breakfast					
Rice cereal	✓				
Lower-fat milk or lower-fat yogurt		✓			
Pear or banana			✓		
Raspberry tea					
Snack					
Oat bran bread	✓				
1 boiled egg					✓
Blueberry tea					
Lunch					
Roast chicken					✓
Whole-grain bread	✓				
Low-fat dressing					
Endive lettuce and thin-sliced avocado				✓	
Mango tea					
Snack					
Low-fat cottage cheese		✓			
Low-fat whole wheat crackers	✓				
Cantaloupe			✓		
Dinner					
Fish, poached in low-fat milk		✓			✓
Potato, mashed or baked	✓				
Spinach				✓	
Squash				✓	
Raspberry ginseng tea					
Snack					
Hummus					✓
Oat cakes	✓				
Strawberries			✓		
Frozen yogurt		✓			

7-Day Menus When Pain Is Severe

Day 1: When Pain Is Severe

Breakfast	AM Snack	Lunch	PM Snack	Dinner	Evening Snack
Puffed rice	Low-fat fruit yogurt	Beta power soup*	Low-fat cottage cheese	Taste of the ocean pasta*	Strawberries
Milk: 1% or 2%		Chicken sandwich on whole-grain bread	Whole wheat biscuits	Beta blend*	Low-fat vanilla pudding
Blueberries		Lettuce or cucumber		Green peas	
Oatmeal bread		Canned pears		Whole-grain bread or roll	
Egg white omelet					
Strawberry tea		Mango tea		Apple spice tea	

Day 2: When Pain Is Severe

Breakfast	AM Snack	Lunch	PM Snack	Dinner	Evening Snack
Oat cereal	1/2 tuna sandwich	Super soothing vegetable stock*	Easy applesauce*	Roast beef	Berry cherry smoothie*
Milk: 1% or 2%		Green salad or cucumbers with oil	Plain or vanilla yogurt	Norma's potato salad*	
Pear nectar		Grilled chicken breast		Green salad, shredded carrots, or green beans	
Flaxseed bread		Whole-grain bread		Grilled zucchini	
Egg: one poached					
Raspberry tea		Blueberry tea	Mango tea		

Asterisks (*) indicate recipes you can find in Part 2: Recipes for Chronic Heartburn and Acid Reflux.

Day 3: When Pain Is Severe

Breakfast	AM Snack	Lunch	PM Snack	Dinner	Evening Snack
Whole wheat cereal	Chopped egg sandwich	Quick and easy green pea soup*	Hummus*	Roast chicken	Fruity splash*
Milk: 1% or 2%		Tuna sandwich on whole-grain bread with baby spinach leaves	Whole-grain pita bread pieces	Brown rice with toasted pine nuts	
Canned plums		Carrot or cucumber sticks	Fruit cocktail	Green peas and water chestnuts	
Oatmeal bread		Creamy coleslaw*		Raw carrots	
Low-fat cheese				Flaxseed bread	
Ginger tea		Strawberry tea		Green tea	

Day 4: When Pain Is Severe

Breakfast	AM Snack	Lunch	PM Snack	Dinner	Evening Snack
Wild berry juice	Low-fat fruit yogurt	Fennel soup*	Whole-grain pita bread	Breaded veal cutlets*	Oatmeal raisin cookies*
Whole wheat cereal		Salmon sandwich on whole-grain bread	Spinach dip*	Boiled potatoes	Milk: 1% or 2%
Milk: 1% or 2%		Lettuce or cucumber		Spinach and strawberry salad with olive oil	
Egg-white omelet		Crimson sunset juice*			
Flaxseed bread					
Apple spice tea		Strawberry tea		Raspberry tea	

Asterisks (*) indicate recipes you can find in Part 2: Recipes for Chronic Heartburn and Acid Reflux.

Day 5: When Pain Is Severe

Breakfast	AM Snack	Lunch	PM Snack	Dinner	Evening Snack
Blueberry juice	Cantaloupe	Lentil soup*	Chicken salad pinwheels*	Beef and Asian vegetable stir fry*	Summer scorcher smoothie*
Oat bran cereal	Low-fat cottage cheese	Baked macaroni and cheese*		Steamed rice	
Milk: 1% or 2%		Carrot and cucumber sticks			
7-grain bread		Flaxseed bread			
1 poached egg					
Strawberry tea		Blueberry tea		Ginger tea	

Day 6: When Pain Is Severe

Breakfast	AM Snack	Lunch	PM Snack	Dinner	Evening Snack
Mixed grain crispy cereal	Easy applesauce*	Chicken noodle soup*	Pita bread	Mango chicken*	Refreshing melon smoothie*
Milk: 1% or 2%	Plain or vanilla yogurt	Grilled cheese sandwich*	Spinach dip*	Oven-roasted potatoes*	
Canned apricots		Vegetable spring rolls*		Baked butternut squash*	
Applesauce-bran muffins*				Waldorf salad*	
Low-fat cheese					
Fruit tea		Mango tea		Raspberry tea	

Asterisks (*) indicate recipes you can find in Part 2: Recipes for Chronic Heartburn and Acid Reflux.

Day 7: When Pain Is Severe

Breakfast	AM Snack	Lunch	PM Snack	Dinner	Evening Snack
Fruity oatmeal*	Low-fat cheese	Russian-style borscht*	Pita bread	Stuffed sole fillets with artichoke dressing*	Sunset smoothie*
Whole-grain toast	Whole-grain crackers	Chicken meatballs*	Hummus*	Mediterranean vegetable hot pot*	
		Brown rice		Flaxseed bread	
		Moroccan-style carrot salad*			
Blueberry tea		Ginger tea		Raspberry tea	

Asterisks (*) indicate recipes you can find in Part 2: Recipes for Chronic Heartburn and Acid Reflux.

Step 2: Meal Plans When Pain Is Coming under Control

As pain starts to come under control, more food choices can be introduced. The menu that follows provides examples incorporating more foods.

Meals	Food Groups				
	Grains, cereals, rice, pasta, starches	Milk, milk products	Fruits	Vegetables	Meats, meat substitutes, legumes, beans, nuts
Breakfast					
Wheat or oat bran cereal	✓				
Lower-fat milk or lower-fat yogurt		✓			
Cherries and blueberries			✓		
Tea					

Meals	Food Groups				
	Grains, cereals, rice, pasta, starches	Milk, milk products	Fruits	Vegetables	Meats, meat substitutes, legumes, beans, nuts
Snack					
Oat bran bread or muffin	✓				
Low-fat cottage cheese		✓			
Blueberry tea					
Lunch					
Egg salad sandwich					✓
Whole-grain bread	✓				
Low-fat dressing					
Endive lettuce and thinly sliced cucumber				✓	
Peaches			✓		
Tea					
Snack					
Hummus					✓
Low-fat whole wheat crackers	✓				
Lower-fat vanilla pudding		✓			
Dinner					
Broiled salmon, with herbs					✓
Steamed rice	✓				
Spinach and mushroom salad with olive oil				✓	
Carrots				✓	
Tea					
Snack					
Low-fat cheese		✓			
Whole-grain toast	✓				
Strawberries and frozen yogurt		✓	✓		

7-Day Menus When Pain Is Coming under Control

Day 1: When Pain Is Coming under Control

Breakfast	AM Snack	Lunch	PM Snack	Dinner	Evening Snack
Whole-grain cereal	Low-fat fruit yogurt	Nonna Vertolli's Minestrone*	Pita bread	Baked chicken fingers*	Whole wheat crackers
Milk: 1% or 2%		Veal burgers*	Hummus*	Oven-roasted potatoes*	
Scrambled egg whites with cheese*		Whole wheat rolls		Italian-style Swiss chard*	Chunky Tzatziki spread*
Flaxseed bread toast		Tossed green salad with olive oil		Whole-grain bread or rolls	
Strawberries and blueberries				Baked apple	
Tea		Tea		Tea	

Day 2: When Pain Is Coming under Control

Breakfast	AM Snack	Lunch	PM Snack	Dinner	Evening Snack
Berry cherry smoothie*	Tuna and pita bread	Asian noodle soup*	Low-fat fruit yogurt	Roast chicken	Oatmeal-raisin cookies*
Oatmeal or oat bran cereal		Baked spinach and rice casserole*		Mixed scalloped potatoes*	Fruity splash*
Milk:1% or 2%		Carrot, celery, and cucumber sticks		Chinese broccoli*	
12-grain toast				Jelly salad*	
Low-fat cheese					
Tea		Tea		Tea	

Asterisks (*) indicate recipes you can find in Part 2: Recipes for Chronic Heartburn and Acid Reflux.

Day 3: When Pain Is Coming under Control

Breakfast	AM Snack	Lunch	PM Snack	Dinner	Evening Snack
Refreshing melon smoothie*	Low-fat cream cheese	A taste of Italy soup*	Salmon sandwich on whole wheat bread	Pork tenderloin with dried fruit*	Crimson sunset juice*
Whole-grain cereal: oats, dry flaxseed, whole wheat	Whole-grain crackers	Mediterranean meatball stew*		Oven-roasted potatoes*	
Milk: 1% or 2%		Tossed green salad with olive oil		Beta blend*	
Flaxseed bread				Just peachy cake*	
Hummus*					
Tea		Tea		Tea	

Day 4: When Pain Is Coming under Control

Breakfast	AM Snack	Lunch	PM Snack	Dinner	Evening Snack
Refreshing fruit blend*	Low-fat fruit yogurt and granola	Creamy potato soup*	Crispy pita triangles*	Grilled tuna steaks with fennel sauce*	Berry cherry smoothie*
Grilled cheese sandwich: low-fat cheese on multigrain bread		Egg salad sandwich on flaxseed bread	Caribbean Fiesta dip*	Brown rice with toasted slivered almonds	
		Carrots, cucumber, and celery sticks		Spinach with raisins*	
				Melon	
Tea		Tea		Tea	

Asterisks (*) indicate recipes you can find in Part 2: Recipes for Chronic Heartburn and Acid Reflux.

Day 5: When Pain Is Coming under Control

Breakfast	AM Snack	Lunch	PM Snack	Dinner	Evening Snack
Fruity oatmeal*	Whole-grain crackers	Apple-carrot-cilantro juice*	Chicken salad pinwheels*	Taste of the Orient salmon*	Strawberries and angel food cake
Strawberries	Low-fat cottage cheese	Middle Eastern pitas*		Baked spinach and rice casserole*	
Flaxseed bread toast		Couscous salad*		Green peas	
Low-fat cheese		Berries and melon		Vanilla yogurt	
Tea		Tea		Tea	

Day 6: When Pain Is Coming under Control

Breakfast	AM Snack	Lunch	PM Snack	Dinner	Evening Snack
Blueberry juice	Oatcakes	Beta power soup*	Fruit yogurt	Hearty veal stew*	Sherbet
Asparagus and mushroom fritatta*	Berries	Chicken with rice*		Mashed sweet potatoes	Melon
Oat bran or flaxseed bread toast		Mixed green salad with olive oil		Waldorf salad*	Milk: 1% or 2%
		Whole-grain bread or rolls		Italian bread	
Tea		Tea		Tea	

Asterisks (*) indicate recipes you can find in Part 2: Recipes for Chronic Heartburn and Acid Reflux.

Day 7: When Pain Is Coming under Control

Breakfast	AM Snack	Lunch	PM Snack	Dinner	Evening Snack
Sunset smoothie*	Fruit yogurt	Fishy rice*	Crispy pita triangles*	Crab chowder*	Refreshing melon smoothie*
Smoked turkey breast frittata*		Creamy coleslaw*	Low-fat cheese	Mango chicken*	
Oat bran or oatmeal bread toast		Crunchy raw vegetables		Baked potato	
		Whole wheat rolls		Roasted zucchini and eggplant	
Tea		Tea		Tea	

Asterisks (*) indicate recipes you can find in Part 2: Recipes for Chronic Heartburn and Acid Reflux.

Step 3: Meal Plans When Pain Is Minimal

Once chronic heartburn and acid reflux symptoms have been brought under control with medications, most people can introduce many more foods. The sample menu provided illustrates ideas on planning for a regimen with fewer restrictions.

Meals	Food Groups				
	Grains, cereals, rice, pasta, starches	Milk, milk products	Fruits	Vegetables	Meats, meat substitutes, legumes, beans, nuts
Breakfast					
Whole-grain wheat or oat cereal	✓				
Lower-fat milk or lower-fat yogurt		✓			
Peaches			✓		
Tea					

Meals	Food Groups				
	Grains, cereals, rice, pasta, starches	Milk, milk products	Fruits	Vegetables	Meats, meat substitutes, legumes, beans, nuts
Snack					
Oat bran bread	✓				
Tuna salad					✓
Lettuce and cucumber				✓	
Tea					
Lunch					
Chicken and vegetable soup				✓	
Broiled salmon with dill					✓
Whole-grain pasta with pesto sauce	✓				
Mixed salad greens and thinly sliced red onions, zucchini and olive oil				✓	
Tea					
Snack					
Low-fat cottage cheese		✓			
Low-fat whole wheat crackers	✓				
Blueberries			✓		
Dinner					
Roast beef					✓
Baked potato	✓				
Steamed broccoli				✓	
Green peas				✓	
Tea					
Snack					
Sliced egg					✓
Whole-grain bread	✓				
Endive and cucumber				✓	
Strawberries and yogurt		✓	✓		

7-Day Menus When Pain Is Minimal

Day 1: When Pain Is Minimal

Breakfast	AM Snack	Lunch	PM Snack	Dinner	Evening Snack
Fruity splash*	Fruit yogurt	Mexican-style black bean soup*	Whole grain crackers	Turkey meatloaf with mushroom gravy*	Chunky tzatziki spread*
Whole-grain wheat or oat cereal	Oatmeal-raisin cookies*	Pasta with green peas*	Salmon-stuffed deviled eggs*	Red-skinned potatoes, roasted	Crispy pita triangles*
Milk: 1% or 2%		Garden salad: lettuce, onion, cucumber, and peppers with olive oil		Green beans and peas	Sorbet
Flaxseed bread toast				Whole-grain bread	
Nut butter: 1 tbsp (15 mL)				Fresh fruit	
Tea		Tea		Tea	

Day 2: When Pain Is Minimal

Breakfast	AM Snack	Lunch	PM Snack	Dinner	Evening Snack
Berries	Fruit yogurt	Chicken meatballs*	Whole-grain crackers	Baked salmon	Refreshing melon smoothie*
Whole-grain dry cereal		Stuffed red peppers*	Low-fat cheese	Green cabbage and potato blend*	
Milk: 1% or 2%		Raw vegetables: carrots, cauliflower, and broccoli		Whole-grain bread or rolls	Spinach with raisins*
	Oat bran bread	Whole-grain bread or rolls		Fresh fruit	
Low-fat cottage cheese					
Tea		Tea		Tea	

Asterisks (*) indicate recipes you can find in Part 2: Recipes for Chronic Heartburn and Acid Reflux.

Day 3: When Pain Is Minimal

Breakfast	AM Snack	Lunch	PM Snack	Dinner	Evening Snack
Mango juice	Easy applesauce*	Apple-carrot-cilantro juice*	Raw vegetables	Turkey meatloaf*	Fruit sorbet
Whole-grain cereal	Vanilla yogurt	Tuna pizza melt*	Spinach dip*	Mixed scalloped potatoes*	Melon
Milk: 1% or 2%		Stuffed red peppers*		Chinese broccoli*	
Flaxseed bread					
Hummus*					
Tea		Tea		Tea	

Day 4: When Pain Is Minimal

Breakfast	AM Snack	Lunch	PM Snack	Dinner	Evening Snack
Fresh melon	Chopped egg sandwich	Truly Canadian split pea soup*	Fruit yogurt	Grilled chicken	Crimson sunset juice*
Whole-grain cereal		Salmon sandwich on whole-grain bread	Jam squares*	Steamed brown rice	Baked potato chips
Milk: 1% or 2%		Raw vegetables: fennel, green beans, and peppers		Beta blend*	
Low-fat cheese on whole-grain bread		Ranch dipping sauce*		Whole-grain bread or rolls	
Tea		Tea		Tea	

Asterisks (*) indicate recipes you can find in Part 2: Recipes for Chronic Heartburn and Acid Reflux.

Day 5: When Pain Is Minimal

Breakfast	AM Snack	Lunch	PM Snack	Dinner	Evening Snack
Mixed fruit	Tuna salad sandwich	Chicken noodle soup*	Raw vegetables	Hamburgers	Berry cherry smoothie*
Whole-grain cereal		Middle Eastern pitas*	Roasted red pepper party dip*	Whole-grain buns	
Milk: 1% or 2%		Spinach with strawberries with olive oil		Creamy coleslaw*	
Whole-grain bread or toast		Fresh fruit		Garden salad with olive oil	
Low-fat cheese					
Tea		Tea		Tea	

Day 6: When Pain Is Minimal

Breakfast	AM Snack	Lunch	PM Snack	Dinner	Evening Snack
Black currant juice	Whole-grain crackers	A taste of Italy soup*	Cool as a cucumber snacks*	Fishy rice*	Summer scorcher smoothie*
Whole-grain cereal	Caribbean fiesta dip*	Swiss chard pizza roll*		Baked butternut squash*	
Milk: 1% or 2%		Garden salad with olive oil		Carrots and green beans	
Scrambled egg whites with cheese*		Cold cuts		Whole-grain bread or rolls	
Whole-grain bread or toast		Fresh fruit			
Tea		Tea		Tea	

Asterisks (*) indicate recipes you can find in Part 2: Recipes for Chronic Heartburn and Acid Reflux.

Breakfast	AM Snack	Lunch	PM Snack	Dinner	Evening Snack
Mango juice	Applesauce-bran muffins*	Winter warming soup*	Graham cracker delight*	Grilled chicken with pesto*	Sorbet
Smoked salmon and vegetable omelet	Fruit yogurt	Asparagus and mushroom frittata*		Artichoke and potato stew*	Fresh fruit
Whole-grain bread or toast		Raw vegetables		Green salad with olive oil	
Hummus*		Ranch dipping sauce*		Whole-grain bread or rolls	
Tea		Tea		Tea	

Asterisks (*) indicate recipes you can find in Part 2: Recipes for Chronic Heartburn and Acid Reflux.

Suggested Grocery List

Now that you're more familiar with what people with acid reflux should and should not eat, it's time to put your diet plan into action. The next step may require replacing what's currently in your refrigerator and pantry with foods that will cause you little or no discomfort. Here's a list of the foods that should be well tolerated that you can purchase at grocery stores. This is just an overview of what to look for when shopping; not all foods available for purchase are mentioned here.

Grain Products

- ❏ Couscous, bulgur, and other grain products
- ❏ Cream of wheat, cream of rice
- ❏ Oatmeal, oat bran (preferably not instant products)
- ❏ Multigrain cold cereals (preferably high in fiber, and ideally without glucose-fructose oligosaccharide or high-fructose corn syrup as a sweetener; sucralose and maltose are acceptable sugar choices)
- ❏ Pasta (preferably whole wheat types)
- ❏ Rice (preferably brown rice, as an additional source of fiber)
- ❏ Whole-grain breads (oat bran, oatmeal, flax, 7-grain, 12-grain)
- ❏ Pitas (whole wheat, flax, cereal grain, and muesli)
- ❏ Wraps (preferably whole-grain)
- ❏ Whole wheat crackers (preferably not greasy or high in fat content)
- ❏ Oatcakes
- ❏ Low-fat granola bars
- ❏ Pretzels

Vegetables and Fruit

Vegetables

- ❏ Artichokes
- ❏ Asparagus
- ❏ Beets and beet greens
- ❏ Belgian endive
- ❏ Carrots
- ❏ Cucumber (peeled)
- ❏ Dark, leafy vegetables, such as baby spinach, spinach, and Swiss chard
- ❏ Fennel/anise
- ❏ Green beans
- ❏ Mushrooms
- ❏ Peas
- ❏ Potatoes, sweet potatoes, yams
- ❏ Radicchio
- ❏ Salad greens
- ❏ Squash (zucchini and winter varieties)
- ❏ If broccoli, Brussels sprouts, cabbage, cauliflower, and turnip are tolerated, include them in meal planning because they are rich in vitamins and minerals

Fruit

- ❏ Apples (not always tolerated raw, but if cooked, as in applesauce, or baked, they are easier to digest)
- ❏ Apricots
- ❏ Berries
- ❏ Canned fruit (except for citrus fruits, such as grapefruit or orange sections)
- ❏ Melons of all types
- ❏ Nectarines
- ❏ Peaches
- ❏ Pears

Milk Products

❏ Skim, 1%, or 2% milk
❏ Low-fat cheese: 4%, 7%, or 17%. Some people will tolerate regular cheeses
❏ Lower-fat cottage cheese (2% or lower fat content)
❏ Lower-fat ice cream; ice milk
❏ Low-fat sour cream
❏ Low-fat yogurt (plain, vanilla, or with fruit)

Meat and Alternatives

❏ Lean or extra-lean red meat
❏ Poultry
❏ Turkey or chicken bacon
❏ Fish (oily varieties, such as mackerel and sardines, might be problematic for some people; other varieties of fish should be tolerated)
❏ Whole eggs or egg whites
❏ Beans (lentils, soybeans, dried peas, chickpeas)
❏ Tofu and tempeh

Desserts

❏ Desserts low in fat and sugar
❏ Low-fat puddings
❏ Sorbets and sherbets

Fats and Oils

❏ Margarines rich in monounsaturated fats (MUFA) and polyunsaturated fats (PUFA): these contain canola and often olive oil; sunflower, safflower, and perhaps corn oils might also be combined with canola or olive oil
❏ Light margarine
❏ Regular or low-fat mayonnaise that does not contain vinegar
❏ Regular or low-fat salad dressings that do not contain vinegar
❏ Avoid palm, palm kernel, and coconut oils because they are all rich in saturated fats

Beverages

❏ Herbal or fruit teas
❏ Fruit juices — preferably unsweetened
❏ Fresh vegetable juices — prepared in juicing facilities or at home in a juicer. Commercially prepared vegetable juices usually contain tomato juice, which is not likely to be tolerated
❏ Bottled water
❏ Non-carbonated beverages
❏ Decaffeinated beverages
❏ Tea is often well tolerated

Seasonings

❏ Gingerroot (if tolerated)
❏ Fresh basil, cilantro, basil, and parsley

Meals Away from Home

When eating away from home, it's important to do some planning in advance. You can maintain control when away from home by being careful about choosing foods and controlling the portions of food that might trigger symptoms. If you drink alcohol, it is best to consume it along with food to reduce the impact it might have.

Eating Out Challenges

Meals away from home can be a challenge for people with chronic heartburn and acid reflux disease for several reasons:

- Social gatherings may include food choices and alcoholic beverages that might not be well tolerated.
- The food available is often rich in fat content, which provides flavor but might not be well tolerated.
- Portion sizes might be larger than usual. Large portion sizes might cause problems, even the day after the social occasion. Restaurant portions tend to be much larger than necessary, so try not to eat any more than you typically would tolerate at home.

In the case of a social occasion with friends or relatives

It is often easy to find out in advance what might be on the menu. Make sure that those who are planning the meal are familiar with the foods and beverages that will cause potential problems. If they are able to provide appropriate substitutes that accommodate your dietary needs, you will have an easy transition from eating at home. Often, however, those providing the meal may not be able to completely accommodate your needs. Taking some of your own food along may work well to give you some control over your choices.

If your job requires that you eat in restaurants on a regular basis

Here are some suggestions for dinner meals that might be well tolerated:

Appetizers

- Clear-type soups, such as vegetable, chicken, beef, or fish broths
- Salads (green leafy types with a small amount of olive or canola oil)
- Pasta or rice salads that do not contain onions, garlic, spices, or tomato products and contain only a small amount of olive or canola oils
- Raw vegetables (carrots, green beans, zucchini, sweet peppers, peeled cucumber, fresh fennel)

Dinner

- Roasted, broiled, or baked meat, poultry, or fish
- Baked, boiled, or mashed potato or rice or pasta without tomato sauce
- Cooked vegetables, such as carrots, green beans, peas, or squash
- Whole-grain bread or roll
- Fruit or neutral fruit juice
- Low-fat cake or cookies as tolerated
- Herbal or fruit tea, or regular tea (if tolerated)

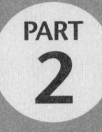

PART 2

Recipes for Chronic Heartburn and Acid Reflux

Preface

"What's for dinner?" This question is undoubtedly a universal one. In many countries around the world, dinner is the most important meal of the day. In the hustle and bustle of everyday life, it is a time for family members to be together while sharing a meal.

For people with chronic heartburn and acid reflux disease, the question of what to eat for dinner is perhaps an even greater concern, simply because of their dietary limitations. Some of the foods that can cause the most pain are readily available in stores and restaurants across North America. While favorites such as French fries, burgers, steak and pizza are indeed appealing to the palate, consuming them can ruin your day or evening if you have acid reflux disease because of the heartburn and accompanying symptoms they often initiate.

Choosing your meals does not have to be stressful. Yes, there are limitations. In order to find relief, you must cut down or completely cut out citrus fruits, tomatoes, an excess of garlic and onions, caffeine, chocolate and high-fat foods. But many alternative low-acid foods can be combined to create great meals. Pasta, for instance, can be enjoyed without the traditional tomato sauce. Grilled vegetables, chicken and pesto sauce make wonderful substitutes. Dips and salad dressings — all of which may seem irreplaceable — can be made with little or no vinegar.

Acid Reflux–Friendly Recipes

The recipes that follow are acid reflux–friendly creations that not only taste good but will make you feel good at the same time.

Not everyone with acid reflux disease will experience discomfort when consuming common trigger foods. You may have a high tolerance for raw onions but be overly sensitive to tomatoes. In these recipes, most of the trigger foods have been eliminated completely to make eating an enjoyable experience for all. The few acidic ingredients that are used appear in small quantities and are to be consumed only if well tolerated.

Living with chronic heartburn, or GERD, does have its disadvantages, but mealtime does not have to be one of them.

Egg and Brunch Dishes

This light meal is perfect for Sunday brunch.

Tip

Canned asparagus tends to be more tender than fresh asparagus.

Asparagus and Mushroom Frittata

- *Preheat broiler*
- *9- to 10-inch (23 to 25 cm) ovenproof nonstick or cast-iron skillet, sprayed with vegetable cooking spray*

1 cup	drained canned chopped asparagus	250 mL
½ cup	drained canned sliced mushrooms	125 mL
1 cup	liquid egg whites	250 mL
2 tbsp	snipped fresh parsley	25 mL
1 tsp	freshly grated Parmesan cheese	5 mL
	Salt	

1. In skillet, heat cooking spray over medium-high heat. Sauté asparagus and mushrooms for 3 to 5 minutes, or until tender-crisp.

2. In a small bowl, beat egg whites, parsley, cheese and salt to taste; pour over vegetables in skillet. Cook, without stirring, for 8 to 10 minutes, or until bottom and sides are firm and top is still slightly runny.

3. Place under preheated broiler, 3 inches (7.5 cm) from the element, for 3 to 5 minutes, or until golden brown. Cut into wedges and serve immediately.

This protein-packed meal is the perfect start to the busy day ahead of you.

Tip

Substitute chicken for turkey, if desired.

Smoked Turkey Breast Frittata

- *Preheat broiler*
- *9- to 10-inch (23 to 25 cm) ovenproof nonstick skillet, sprayed with vegetable cooking spray*

¼ cup	minced red bell pepper	50 mL
2 tbsp	minced green onion (optional, as tolerated)	25 mL
¾ cup	finely chopped smoked turkey breast deli slices	175 mL
1 cup	liquid egg whites	250 mL
	Snipped fresh parsley	
	Salt	

1. In skillet, heat cooking spray over medium-high heat. Sauté red pepper and onions (if using) for 4 to 5 minutes, or until tender. Add turkey breast and cook for 1 minute. Add egg whites and parsley and salt to taste, stirring once. Cook, without stirring, for 8 to 10 minutes, until bottom and sides are firm and top is still slightly runny.

2. Place under preheated broiler, 3 inches (7.5 cm) from the element, for 3 to 5 minutes, until golden brown. Cut into wedges and serve immediately.

Health Tip

This recipe is full of flavor — the sweet peppers and parsley are a great complement to the egg and meat combination. The eggs and turkey are good sources of protein, as well as vitamins and minerals. This frittata should be well tolerated by anyone with chronic heartburn or acid reflux disease.

Using egg whites and eliminating the crust makes these quiches a light addition to your breakfast menu.

Tips

Use canned or bottled roasted red peppers for convenience. They can be found in the canned vegetable section of most grocery stores.

Quiche can be cooked in paper muffin cups if desired.

Make ahead

Place cooled quiche in an airtight container and store in the freezer for 6 to 8 months. Thaw and warm in microwave oven on High for 3 to 4 minutes.

Breakfast Quiche

- *Preheat oven to 350°F (180°C)*
- *6-cup jumbo muffin tin, lightly greased*

10 oz	finely chopped fresh spinach	300 g
1/3 cup	snipped green onions (optional, as tolerated)	75 mL
1 cup	liquid egg whites	250 mL
1/4 cup	diced roasted red bell pepper	50 mL
1 tsp	snipped fresh parsley	5 mL
	Salt	
1/3 cup	shredded mozzarella cheese	75 mL

1. Spray a large skillet with vegetable cooking spray and heat over high heat. Sauté spinach and onions (if using) for 4 to 5 minutes, or until spinach is wilted. Drain.

2. In a medium bowl, beat spinach mixture, egg whites, red pepper, parsley and salt to taste.

3. Divide mixture evenly among 4 muffin cups, filling empty cups with water about ¾ full to prevent tin from warping. Sprinkle cheese lightly over each quiche. Bake in preheated oven for 25 to 30 minutes, or until a knife inserted in the center comes out clean.

If you love scrambled eggs for breakfast, here's a lighter version of a North American favorite.

Scrambled Egg Whites with Cheese

3	egg whites	3
1 tbsp	shredded low-fat Swiss cheese	15 mL
1 tsp	minced fresh parsley	5 mL
	Salt	

1. In a small bowl, beat egg whites with cheese, parsley and salt to taste.

2. Spray a small skillet with vegetable cooking spray and heat over medium-high heat. Cook egg white mixture, stirring, for 4 to 5 minutes, or until eggs are no longer runny.

Variation: Substitute soy cheese alternative for the Swiss cheese.

These are healthier than the burritos you would find at most fast food chains and take less than 10 minutes to make.

Tip

For extra protein, add ¼ cup (50 mL) chopped lean deli slices in Step 1.

Breakfast Burritos

½ cup	liquid egg whites, beaten	125 mL
½ cup	chopped red bell pepper	125 mL
¼ cup	shredded lettuce	50 mL
¼ cup	shredded low-fat cheese (such as Swiss or mozzarella)	50 mL
	Salt	
2	whole wheat flour tortillas	2

1. Spray a small skillet with vegetable cooking spray and heat over medium-high heat. Cook egg whites and pepper, stirring, for 5 to 7 minutes, or until eggs are no longer runny.

2. In a small bowl, combine egg white mixture, lettuce, cheese and salt to taste.

3. Divide egg white mixture evenly between tortillas. Roll each wrap into a packet to enclose the filling.

Hash browns are a popular North American breakfast food that people with acid reflux can't often indulge in. These patties are baked and are dipped in egg whites, therefore eliminating some of the triggers that can cause digestive distress.

Breakfast Potato Patties

- *Preheat oven to 400°F (200°C)*
- *Baking sheet, lined with foil and greased*

3 cups	grated peeled potatoes	750 mL
1/2 cup	grated peeled carrots	125 mL
2 tbsp	grated onion (optional, as tolerated)	25 mL
1/3 cup	liquid egg whites	75 mL
1/4 cup	all-purpose flour	50 mL
1 tbsp	canola oil	15 mL
1 tbsp	snipped fresh parsley	15 mL
1/4 tsp	baking powder	1 mL
	Salt	

1. In a colander, drain potatoes, carrots and onion (if using). Using your hands, squeeze out excess liquid.

2. In a large bowl, beat egg whites, flour, oil, parsley, baking powder and salt to taste. Stir in grated vegetables and mix thoroughly. Form into six 2-inch (5 cm) round patties.

3. Place on prepared baking sheet and bake in preheated oven for 9 to 10 minutes, or until browned on top. Flip patties and bake for 9 to 10 minutes, or until browned.

Variation: Add 1/2 tsp (2 mL) chopped fresh rosemary.

French Toast

1 tbsp	light margarine	15 mL
1/2 cup	liquid egg whites	125 mL
1/2 cup	skim milk or lactose-free skim milk	125 mL
2 tsp	lightly packed brown sugar	10 mL
1/2 tsp	ground cinnamon	2 mL
1/2 tsp	vanilla	2 mL
4	slices whole wheat bread	4

1. In a large skillet, melt margarine over medium-high heat.
2. Meanwhile, in a shallow bowl, beat egg whites, milk, brown sugar, cinnamon and vanilla.
3. Dip each piece of bread in egg white mixture, turning to coat both sides. Immediately drop bread onto the hot skillet and cook, turning once or twice to cook evenly on both sides, for 2 to 3 minutes per side, or until browned.

Fruity Oatmeal

2/3 cup	quick-cooking rolled oats	150 mL
1/2 cup	drained canned peach halves, finely sliced	125 mL
3 tbsp	lightly packed brown sugar	45 mL
1 tsp	liquid honey	5 mL
1/2 tsp	ground cinnamon	2 mL

1. In a medium saucepan, bring 1 1/2 cups (375 mL) water to a boil over high heat. Add oats, reduce heat to medium-high and cook, stirring, for 3 minutes. Stir in peaches, brown sugar, honey and cinnamon; cook, stirring, for 3 to 4 minutes, or until water has been absorbed.

Creamy Rice Pudding

Using less sugar and low-fat milk makes this a more healthful addition to your breakfast menu.

Tips

Do not leave to simmer. Stir frequently to avoid sticking and burning.

Add more liquid as needed.

4 cups	1% milk or lactose-free 1% milk, divided	1 L
1 cup	short-grain white rice	250 mL
2 tbsp	lightly packed brown sugar	25 mL
½ tsp	ground cinnamon	2 mL
½ tsp	salt	2 mL
½ tsp	vanilla	2 mL
¾ cup	golden raisins	175 mL

1. In a medium saucepan, heat 3 cups (750 mL) of the milk over medium heat. Add rice, brown sugar, cinnamon, salt and vanilla; Reduce heat and simmer, stirring frequently, for 25 to 30 minutes, gradually adding the remaining milk as rice starts to absorb liquid, until rice is almost tender. Stir in raisins and simmer until rice is tender and liquid is absorbed, about 15 minutes.

Variation: Use long-grain rice for a less creamy rice pudding.

Health Tip

What a nutrient-rich, tasty choice! A touch of cinnamon with brown sugar and raisins provides a complementary flavor and texture to the rice. This recipe is a great source of protein, soluble fiber, calcium and iron. It's easy for people of all ages to digest. If you do not tolerate milk, you can try substituting lactose-reduced milk or soy milk.

Appetizers

Traditional hummus can often be a trial for those with acid reflux due to its garlic and oil content. I have significantly reduced both of these ingredients, making it an acid reflux–friendly treat.

Tips

Tahini is a thick, creamy paste made from sesame seeds.

Serve as a tasty spread for pita bread or as a dip with vegetables.

Make ahead

Spoon into an airtight container and store in the refrigerator for up to 3 days.

Hummus

2	cans (each 19 oz/540 mL) chickpeas, drained and rinsed	2
¼ cup	warm water	50 mL
2 tbsp	tahini (optional)	25 mL
¼ tsp	onion powder (optional, as tolerated)	1 mL
	Salt	
	Snipped fresh parsley	
1 tbsp	extra-virgin olive oil	15 mL
1	whole clove garlic	1

1. In a food processor, grind chickpeas, water, tahini (if using), onion powder (if using) and salt and parsley to taste until chunky. Add oil and continue grinding until mixture is smooth.

2. Transfer to a serving bowl and stir in garlic. Cover and refrigerate for 4 to 5 hours to allow flavors to blend. Remove garlic clove before serving.

Health Tip

This hummus can be readily digested and is well tolerated by people with acid reflux. It's a great snack with bread or crackers, as an appetizer or as part of a main meal.

The mild flavor of this hummus is highlighted by parsley and a touch of garlic. It is a rich source of protein, soluble fiber and a variety of minerals and vitamins.

Spinach Dip

Makes ¾ cup (175 mL)

This light dip is a great way to entice kids to eat their greens.

Tips

Sauté 2 cups (500 mL) raw spinach in a skillet sprayed with vegetable cooking spray or in 1 tsp (5 mL) canola oil over high heat until tender. Let cool before making dip.

Serve with pumpernickel bread or raw veggies.

Make ahead

Spoon into an airtight container and store in the refrigerator for up to 4 days.

½ cup	finely chopped cooked spinach	125 mL
¼ cup	low-fat plain yogurt	50 mL
1 tsp	fat-free mayonnaise-style sauce	5 mL
	Salt	

1. In a small bowl, combine spinach, yogurt, mayonnaise and salt to taste. Cover and refrigerate for at least 1 hour to allow flavors to blend.

Caribbean Fiesta Dip

Makes 1 cup (250 mL)

This sweet-tasting dip is a nice alternative to plum sauce, which is often loaded with vinegar. Papaya, a revered digestive aid, is an added bonus.

Tip

Serve with chicken fingers or spring rolls.

Make ahead

Spoon into an airtight container and store in the refrigerator for up to 3 days.

1 cup	drained canned mango slices	250 mL
1 cup	drained canned papaya slices	250 mL
1 tbsp	liquid honey	15 mL

1. In a blender or food processor, on high speed, purée mango, papaya and honey until smooth.

Roasted Red Pepper Party Dip

This dip is always a hit with guests. Serve with pita bread or whole wheat crackers for a great party appetizer.

Tips

You may need to drain the peppers again after they go through the food processor.

The mixture will thicken as it chills.

Make ahead

Spoon into an airtight container and store in the refrigerator for up to 4 days.

2 cups	roasted red bell peppers, drained	500 mL
½ cup	low-fat plain yogurt	125 mL
Pinch	garlic powder (optional, as tolerated)	Pinch
	Snipped fresh parsley	
	Salt	

1. In a food processor, finely chop peppers (the consistency should be chunky). Transfer to a bowl and stir in yogurt, garlic powder (if using) and parsley and salt to taste until smooth. Cover and refrigerate for at least 1 hour to allow flavors to blend.

Chunky Tzatziki Spread

This light spread is adapted from a recipe used in traditional Greek cuisine.

Tip

Serve with lower-fat tortilla chips, raw veggies or pita triangles.

Make ahead

Spoon into an airtight container and store in the refrigerator for up to 4 days.

½ cup	grated English cucumber	125 mL
¼ cup	fat-free plain yogurt	50 mL
½ tsp	dried dillweed	2 mL
	Snipped fresh parsley	
	Salt	
1	whole garlic clove	1

1. Squeeze grated cucumber in a colander to remove excess liquid.
2. In a small bowl, combine cucumber, yogurt, dill and parsley and salt to taste. Stir in garlic clove, cover and refrigerate for 4 to 5 hours to allow flavors to blend. Remove garlic clove before serving.

Variation: For a creamy cucumber salad dressing, reduce the amount of grated cucumber to taste.

Ranch Dipping Sauce

Traditional ranch dressing is often loaded with garlic and onions. Reducing both of these ingredients makes it better suited for those with acid reflux.

1 cup	fat-free sour cream	250 mL
2 tbsp	minced red bell pepper	25 mL
1 tsp	dried dillweed	5 mL
1 tsp	snipped fresh chives (optional)	5 mL
	Salt	

Tips

Serve with chicken fingers or raw veggies.

Using dillweed eliminates the need for vinegar in this dip. Dill has a similar taste to vinegar, without the acidity.

Make ahead

Spoon into an airtight container and store in the refrigerator for up to 4 days.

1. In a small bowl, combine sour cream, red pepper, dill, chives (if using) and salt to taste. Cover and refrigerate for at least 1 hour to allow flavors to blend.

Variation: Use low-fat plain yogurt, if preferred, in place of the sour cream.

Makes 12 appetizers

Five-Minute Meat-on-a-Stick Appetizers

This recipe is perfect for when unexpected visitors arrive at your doorstep. Increase ingredients as needed.

12	low-fat breadsticks	12
6	extra-lean turkey breast deli slices	6
6	extra-lean chicken breast deli slices	6
	Romaine lettuce	

1. Wrap individual deli slices around each breadstick. Serve on beds of Romaine lettuce.

Variation: Substitute smoked salmon or extra-lean smoked ham deli slices.

Shrimp Canapés

Light margarine and fat-free mayonnaise help make these canapés less fattening than typical restaurant appetizers.

- *Preheat broiler*
- *Baking sheet, ungreased*

¼ cup	shredded low-fat mozzarella cheese	50 mL
2 tbsp	light margarine, softened	25 mL
2 tsp	fat-free mayonnaise	10 mL
½ tsp	dried parsley	2 mL
Pinch	garlic powder (optional, as tolerated)	Pinch
	Salt	
½ cup	drained salad shrimp	125 mL
4	whole wheat English muffins, halved	4

1. In a medium bowl, combine cheese, margarine, mayonnaise, parsley, garlic powder (if using) and salt to taste until blended. Add shrimp and spread evenly over English muffin halves.

2. Place on baking sheet and broil for 3 to 4 minutes, or until cheese has melted. Cut into quarters and serve warm.

> **Variations:** Use toast instead of English muffins.
>
> Try using canned crab meat instead of shrimp.

Makes 12 appetizers

Eliminating the egg yolks in this appetizer makes it less rich than the traditional recipe.

Make ahead

Place in an airtight container and store in the refrigerator for up to 3 days.

Salmon-Stuffed Deviled Eggs

6	hard-cooked eggs	6
1 cup	drained canned salmon, skin and bones removed	250 mL
3 tbsp	fat-free sour cream	45 mL
1 tsp	snipped fresh dill	5 mL
¼ tsp	paprika	1 mL
	Salt	

1. Slice eggs in half lengthwise and scoop out the yolks. Discard yolks.

2. In a small bowl, combine salmon, sour cream, dill, paprika and salt to taste.

3. Stuff egg whites with salmon mixture. Cover and refrigerate for at least 1 hour to allow flavors to blend.

Variations: Try fat-free mayonnaise instead of sour cream.

If serving a large number of guests, try making a variety of canned tuna, crab and salmon fillings.

 Health Tip

The mild flavor of egg whites has been combined with several complementary ingredients. Salmon, sour cream, paprika, salt and dill all work together with the egg to create an interesting appetizer or light meal. This recipe is a great source of protein and minerals. If sour cream is used, calcium will be present, and if egg yolks are used, it becomes a significant source of iron as well. It's a recipe that should be well tolerated if you are experiencing heartburn.

Chicken Salad Pinwheels

Your guests will be sure to appreciate this quick and tasty appetizer.

Tips

Recipe can easily be doubled.

To cook chicken breasts, grill for 8 to 10 minutes per side or simmer in broth for 30 to 40 minutes, until chicken has reached an internal temperature of 170°F (75°C) and is no longer pink inside.

2	boneless skinless chicken breasts (about ½ lb/250 g), cooked, cooled and shredded	2
¼ cup	fat-free mayonnaise	50 mL
2 tbsp	minced red bell pepper	25 mL
1 tbsp	snipped fresh parsley	15 mL
	Salt	
2	spinach-flavored flour tortillas	2
	Romaine lettuce	

1. In a small bowl, combine chicken, mayonnaise, red pepper, parsley and salt to taste.

2. Spread half of mixture evenly over each tortilla. Begin rolling wraps from the edge closest to you, jelly-roll style, using your fingers to hold filling in place. Cover and refrigerate for 2 to 3 hours, or until set.

3. Place rolls seam side down on a cutting board and cut into 1-inch (2.5 cm) pieces. Place on beds of Romaine lettuce.

Variation: When serving a large number of guests, try making a variety of pinwheels, using tuna and salmon salad as well as chicken salad. For tuna or salmon salad, substitute 1 cup (250 mL) drained tuna or salmon for the chicken.

Using a small amount of lower-fat cheese goes a long way toward making these appetizers lighter and healthier than what you'd find on a restaurant menu.

Tip

This recipe can easily be doubled.

Baked Mushroom Caps

- *Preheat oven to 375°F (190°C)*
- *Baking sheet, lightly greased*

¼ cup	low-fat shredded Swiss cheese	50 mL
3 tbsp	seasoned dry bread crumbs	45 mL
1 tsp	dried parsley	5 mL
	Salt	
6	jumbo mushrooms	6

1. In a small bowl, combine cheese, bread crumbs, parsley and salt to taste.
2. Remove stems from mushrooms. Using a spoon, scrape out gills from cap, making a cavity for filling. Divide the cheese mixture evenly among the mushroom caps, heaping as necessary.
3. Place on prepared baking sheet and bake in preheated oven for 15 to 20 minutes, or until cheese has melted and mushrooms are tender.

Makes 48 appetizers

My significant other introduced me to these delightful morsels. Serve when guests arrive, or enjoy as a hot afternoon snack.

Tips

If using as an appetizer, serve on beds of baby spinach.

Peel cucumbers if you find the skin difficult to digest.

Cool as a Cucumber Snacks

2	large English cucumbers	2
24	extra-lean turkey and chicken deli slices, sliced in half	24

1. Slice cucumbers into ½-inch (1 cm) thick slices.
2. Wrap a deli slice around each cucumber slice and secure with a toothpick.

Crispy Pita Triangles

These triangles are a nice alternative to garlic bread. They're lighter, with only a hint of garlic flavor.

- *Preheat oven to 350°F (180°C)*
- *Baking sheet, ungreased*

1 tbsp	dried parsley	15 mL
1 tsp	dried basil	5 mL
½ tsp	freshly grated Romano or Parmesan cheese	2 mL
¼ tsp	garlic powder (optional, as tolerated)	1 mL
3	large pitas (any kind), sliced into 24 triangles	3

1. Sprinkle parsley, basil, cheese and garlic powder (if using) on pita triangles. Place on baking sheet in a single layer and bake in preheated oven for 5 minutes, or to desired crispness.

Variation: Use spinach-flavored flour tortillas instead of pitas, if desired.

➡ Health Tip

This is a flavorful version of pita bread, a great combination with dips and spreads. The cheese and hint of garlic blend well with the herbs, all of which are then further enhanced by toasting in the oven to a crisp texture. The key nutrients are carbohydrates and a touch of protein, with some B vitamins. This recipe should be tolerated well if you have heartburn.

Pair this savory appetizer
with minestrone for a
real Sicilian feast!

Sicilian Spinach Bread

• *Preheat oven to 375°F (190°C)*

1 tbsp	extra-virgin olive oil	15 mL
10 oz	fresh spinach, trimmed and finely chopped	300 g
1/3 cup	finely chopped green onions (as tolerated)	75 mL
1/2 tsp	garlic powder (optional, as tolerated)	2 mL
	Salt	
1	large French baguette	1
2 tbsp	light margarine	25 mL
1/2 cup	low-fat shredded mozzarella cheese	125 mL

1. In a medium saucepan, heat oil over high heat. Sauté spinach, onions (if using), garlic powder (if using) and salt to taste for 5 to 7 minutes, or until wilted. Remove from heat.

2. Slice baguette in half lengthwise. Spread margarine and spinach mixture over each half. Sprinkle with cheese.

3. Sandwich the two halves with topping pressed together and wrap in foil. Bake in preheated oven for 10 minutes. Spread the foil open and bake for 5 minutes longer, or until bread is hot. Cut into 2-inch (5 cm) thick slices.

People with acid reflux can reap the benefits of pesto made from fresh herbs. Basil has a reputation for easing digestive disorders and dispelling gas.

Tip

Use more pesto if desired.

Pesto Crostini

- *Preheat oven to 425°F (220°C)*
- *Baking sheet, lightly greased*

½	large French baguette	½
2	roasted red bell peppers, minced	2
½ cup	Pesto Sauce (see recipe, page 187)	125 mL
2 tbsp	freshly grated Romano cheese	25 mL

1. Slice baguette into 1-inch (2.5 cm) thick slices. Spoon ½ tsp (2 mL) peppers and ½ tsp (2 mL) pesto onto each slice, spreading to cover. Sprinkle with cheese.

2. Place on prepared baking sheet and bake in preheated oven for 2 to 3 minutes, or until browned.

Variation: Add grilled zucchini sliced in matchsticks.

Health Tip

What a taste experience! The crisp texture of the baguette is combined with the soft roasted sweet peppers, the savory touch of cheese and the rich flavor of olive oil. Key nutrients include B vitamins and a variety of minerals and carbohydrates from the bread. The combination of flavors and textures in this recipe provides lots of taste appeal and should be tolerated if you have heartburn and acid reflux.

Soups

This soup base is the ultimate comfort food, sure to leave you feeling warm and cozy inside.

Tips

Cut up the cooked vegetables and serve with steamed rice.

Use the cooked chicken breasts to make Chicken Salad Pinwheels (see recipe, page 130).

Make ahead

Ladle into an airtight container and store in the refrigerator for up to 4 days or in the freezer for up to 3 months.

Feel Better Chicken Stock

1 lb	chicken breasts (bone-in), skin removed and fat trimmed	500 g
4	stalks celery, with leaves	4
4	carrots, peeled and halved	4
2	onions (optional, as tolerated)	2
2	bay leaves	2
1	parsnip, peeled and halved	1
	Fresh parsley	
	Salt	

1. Place chicken, celery, carrots, onions (if using), bay leaves, parsnip and parsley and salt to taste in a large stockpot and add 12 cups (3 L) of water, or enough to fully cover ingredients. Bring to a boil over high heat. Reduce heat to medium-low and simmer, partially covered, for $1\frac{1}{2}$ hours, until stock is flavorful and liquid is reduced by about one-quarter. Strain stock through a fine-mesh sieve set over a large bowl. (Chicken and vegetables may be saved for use in other recipes.)

Health Tip

Does chicken soup have a medicinal quality? Why don't you try it! This soup is mild and tasty with hints of flavors from combining chicken, bay leaves, parsley, salt, celery, carrots, onions and parsnips. The nutritional benefits from this recipe include moderate amounts of salt and potassium. If you have heartburn, you should be able to tolerate this soup.

Super Soothing Vegetable Stock

This light stock serves well as a base for hearty vegetable soups.

If tolerated, add a sweet yellow tomato, quartered and seeded. Yellow tomatoes have less acid than regular varieties.

Make ahead

Ladle into an airtight container and store in the refrigerator for up to 4 days or in the freezer for up to 3 months.

3	carrots, peeled and halved	3
3	stalks celery, with leaves	3
2	potatoes	2
2	bay leaves	2
1	onion (optional, as tolerated)	1
1	parsnip, peeled and halved	1
	Fresh parsley	
	Salt	

1. Place 10 cups (2.5 L) water, carrots, celery, potatoes, bay leaves, onion, parsnip and parsley and salt to taste in a large stockpot. Bring to a boil over high heat. Reduce heat to medium-low and simmer, partially covered, for $1\frac{1}{2}$ hours, until stock is flavorful and liquid is reduced by one-fifth. Strain broth through a fine-mesh sieve set over a large bowl.

Serves 4 to 6

Winter Warming Soup

This soup is perfect on a cold winter's day. Serve with warm bread.

If frozen turnips are not available, use an equal amount of fresh turnip or rutabaga, peeled and diced. Add with the carrots.

5 cups	vegetable stock (store-bought or see recipe, above)	1.25 L
3	carrots, peeled and finely sliced	3
3	potatoes, peeled and finely sliced	3
2	bay leaves	2
1 cup	finely sliced collard greens (leaves only)	250 mL
2 tbsp	snipped fresh parsley	25 mL
	Salt	
$\frac{1}{2}$ cup	diced frozen turnip	125 mL

1. In a large saucepan, bring stock to a boil over high heat. Add carrots, potatoes, bay leaves, collard greens, parsley and salt to taste. Reduce heat to medium-low and simmer, partially covered, for 30 minutes, until vegetables are tender-crisp. Add turnips and simmer for 10 minutes, until tender. Discard bay leaves.

Beta Power Soup

Tip

If desired, substitute ½-inch (1 cm) piece of gingerroot, peeled and minced, for the ground ginger.

Make ahead

Ladle into an airtight container and store in the refrigerator for up to 4 days or in the freezer for up to 3 months.

2	carrots, peeled and finely sliced	2
4 cups	cubed peeled butternut squash	1 L
3 cups	vegetable stock (store-bought or see recipe, page 137)	750 mL
¼ tsp	ground ginger	1 mL
¼ tsp	onion powder (optional, as tolerated)	1 mL
¼ cup	skim milk or lactose-free skim milk	50 mL
	Snipped fresh cilantro	

1. Spray a large saucepan with vegetable cooking spray and heat over medium-high heat. Sauté carrots and squash for 5 minutes, until tender-crisp. Add stock, ginger and onion powder (if using); bring to a boil. Reduce heat to medium-low and simmer, partially covered, for 30 minutes, or until vegetables are tender. Remove from heat and let cool.

2. Transfer soup to a blender and blend on medium speed until smooth. Return to pot and place over low heat. Stir in milk and cilantro to taste; simmer for 3 to 5 minutes, or until heated through.

Health Tip

Carrots and squash combined with ginger and cilantro in a vegetable stock form the essence of this tasty soup. The vegetables are cooked and then blended into a smooth purée, providing a rich source of the antioxidant vitamin A precursor beta-carotene, as well as other vitamins and minerals. A touch of milk contributes a little protein and calcium to the soup. If you have heartburn and acid reflux, you will find this soup soothing and tasty. If you do not tolerate dairy products, you can substitute lactose-reduced milk or plain soy milk.

This hearty soup is adapted from a popular Italian recipe used frequently in my family. Serve with warm Italian bread for dunking.

Tips

Romano beans are also known as cranberry beans.

Garlic has a very strong flavor and can cause heartburn in those with acid reflux. Cooking with a whole garlic clove adds a nice flavor to the soup, and you don't actually have to consume it.

Make ahead

Ladle into an airtight container and store in the refrigerator for up to 4 days or in the freezer for up to 3 months.

A Taste of Italy Soup

1 tsp	extra-virgin olive oil	5 mL
2	carrots, peeled and finely sliced	2
1	whole clove garlic (optional, as tolerated)	1
4 cups	coarsely chopped escarole	1 L
2½ cups	chicken stock (store-bought or see recipe, page 136)	625 mL
1 tbsp	snipped fresh parsley	15 mL
1 tsp	snipped fresh basil	5 mL
1	can (14 oz/398 mL) romano beans, drained and rinsed	1

1. In a medium saucepan, heat oil over medium-high heat. Sauté carrots and garlic (if using) for 3 to 4 minutes, or until slightly softened. Add escarole, stock, parsley and basil; bring to a boil. Reduce heat to medium-low and simmer, partially covered, for 30 minutes, until vegetables are tender. Add beans and simmer for 5 minutes, until heated through. Discard garlic clove.

> **Variation:** If beans are not well tolerated, substitute two medium potatoes, peeled and diced. Add with the carrots.

Serves 6 to 8

There's nothing like homemade chicken noodle soup to ease your aches and pains.

Tip

If you don't want to use all the chicken, reserve some for chicken salad sandwich filling.

Make ahead

Ladle into an airtight container and store in the refrigerator for up to 4 days or in the freezer for up to 3 months.

Chicken Noodle Soup

2	bay leaves	2
1	onion (optional, as tolerated)	1
1 lb	chicken breasts (bone-in), skins removed and fat trimmed	500 g
	Fresh parsley	
	Salt	
3	large carrots, peeled and cut in $\frac{1}{2}$-inch (1 cm) slices	3
2	stalks celery (with leaves), cut in $\frac{1}{2}$-inch (1 cm) slices	2
6 oz	noodles (any kind)	175 g

1. In a large stock pot, combine 8 cups (2 L) water, bay leaves, onion (if using), chicken and parsley and salt to taste; bring to a boil over high heat. Reduce heat to medium-low and simmer, partially covered, for 1 hour, until chicken is no longer pink inside. Add carrots and celery; simmer for 20 to 25 minutes, or until tender.

2. Meanwhile, bring a medium pot of salted water to a boil over high heat and cook noodles according to package directions. Drain and set aside.

3. Remove chicken, onion and bay leaves from stock pot. Discard onion and bay leaves. De-bone chicken and finely slice. Add back to soup and stir in noodles. Serve immediately.

> **Variation:** Add 1 parsnip, peeled and cut in $\frac{1}{2}$-inch (1 cm) slices, with the celery and carrots.

My grandmother used to make this soup for me when I wasn't feeling well, and now I make it for her.

Tips

Substitute white kidney beans for the romano beans, if preferred.

Onion powder is generally better tolerated than minced onion. Feel free to use $1/2$ cup (125 mL) minced onion, though, if it's well tolerated.

Make ahead

Ladle into an airtight container and store in the refrigerator for up to 4 days or in the freezer for up to 3 months.

Nonna Vertolli's Minestrone

6 cups	chicken stock (store-bought or see recipe, page 136)	1.5 L
2	bay leaves	2
2	carrots, peeled and finely chopped	2
1	stalk celery, finely chopped	1
2 tbsp	snipped fresh parsley	25 mL
$1/4$ tsp	onion powder (optional, as tolerated)	1 mL
3 cups	coarsely chopped fresh spinach	750 mL
1 cup	drained and rinsed canned romano beans	250 mL
$1/2$ cup	star-shaped pasta	125 mL
	Salt	

1. In a large saucepan, bring stock to a boil over high heat. Add bay leaves, carrots, celery, parsley and onion powder (if using). Reduce heat to medium-low and simmer, partially covered, for 30 minutes, until vegetables are tender. Add spinach and beans; simmer for 5 to 10 minutes, or until spinach is wilted.

2. Add pasta and remove from heat, placing the lid firmly on the saucepan. The pasta will take approximately 25 minutes to expand and cook in the hot liquid. Discard bay leaves.

The title says it all. This soup is perfect for no-fuss dinners or lunches.

Tip

If preferred, substitute snipped fresh parsley for the cilantro.

Make ahead

Ladle into an airtight container and store in the refrigerator for up to 4 days or in the freezer for up to 3 months.

Quick and Easy Green Pea Soup

1 tsp	light margarine	5 mL
1	large carrot, peeled and finely sliced	1
1/4 cup	minced red onion (optional, as tolerated)	50 mL
2 cups	thawed frozen sweet peas	500 mL
2 cups	vegetable stock (store-bought or see recipe, page 137)	500 mL
	Snipped fresh cilantro	
	Salt	
1/2 cup	1% milk or lactose-free 1% milk	125 mL

1. In a medium saucepan, melt margarine over medium-high heat. Sauté carrot and onion (if using) for 3 to 5 minutes, or until tender. Add peas, stock and cilantro and salt to taste; bring to a boil. Reduce heat to medium-low and simmer, partially covered, for 15 minutes, until peas are tender. Remove from heat and let cool.

2. Transfer soup to a blender and blend on medium speed until smooth. Return to pot and place over low heat. Gradually stir in milk and simmer for 5 minutes, until heated through.

Health Tip

A great source of nutrients! Frozen peas are the main ingredient in this easy-to-prepare, tasty soup. The peas are a source of soluble and insoluble dietary fiber, protein and a variety of minerals and vitamins. Peas are readily digestible and well tolerated if you have acid reflux problems.

Creamy Potato Soup

This is a light version of a soup traditionally made with heavy cream and an excessive amount of leeks.

1 cup	minced leeks (white and light green parts only)	250 mL
4	large red-skinned potatoes, peeled and diced	4
2	carrots, peeled and finely sliced	2
1	stalk celery, finely sliced	1
3½ cups	vegetable stock (store-bought or see recipe, page 137)	875 mL
2	bay leaves	2
3 tbsp	snipped fresh parsley	45 mL
1 tbsp	snipped fresh basil	15 mL
	Salt	
1 cup	1% milk or lactose-free 1% milk	250 mL

1. Spray a large saucepan with vegetable cooking spray and heat over high heat. Sauté leeks for 2 to 3 minutes, until tender. Add potatoes, carrots and celery; sauté for 2 to 3 minutes, until slightly softened. Add stock, bay leaves, parsley, basil and salt to taste; bring to a boil. Reduce heat to medium low and simmer, partially covered, for 30 to 40 minutes, until vegetables are tender. Remove from heat and gradually stir in milk. Discard bay leaves.

> **Variation:** Add ½ cup (125 mL) fresh or frozen cut green beans with the potatoes.

Fennel Soup

Fennel is a revered digestive aid, making this soup a must on bad heartburn days.

Tip

If using dried white kidney beans, reduce amount to $1/2$ cup (125 mL). Place beans in bowl and cover with water. Let soak overnight. Drain and rinse. In a pot, cover beans with cold water and bring to a boil over high heat. Boil for about 30 minutes, until tender. Drain before adding to soup.

Make ahead

Ladle into an airtight container and store in the refrigerator for up to 4 days or in the freezer for up to 3 months.

5 cups	chicken stock (store-bought or see recipe, page 136)	1.25 L
2	carrots, peeled and finely sliced	2
1	bay leaf	1
3 cups	chopped fennel bulbs	750 mL
3 tbsp	snipped fresh parsley	45 mL
$1/2$ tsp	snipped fresh oregano	2 mL
$1/4$ tsp	onion powder (optional, as tolerated)	1 mL
	Salt	
1 cup	drained and rinsed canned white kidney beans	250 mL

1. In a large saucepan, bring stock to a boil over high heat. Add carrots, bay leaf, fennel, parsley, oregano, onion powder (if using) and salt to taste. Reduce heat to medium-low and simmer, partially covered, for 35 minutes, until vegetables are tender. Add beans and simmer for 10 minutes, until beans are heated through. Discard bay leaf.

➡ Health Tip

Fennel and carrots are the primary vegetables in this soup, combined with kidney beans and fragrant herbs that add an interesting additional flavor. The beans provide a soft texture to complement the firmer texture of the key vegetables. Fennel has a mild licorice-like flavor and is easy to digest, while both vegetables provide an important source of protein, fiber, vitamins, and minerals.

Crab Chowder

This chowder is not as rich and heavy as the traditional New England soup, so it's suitable for people with acid reflux.

3	large potatoes, peeled and chopped	3
2	carrots, peeled and finely sliced	2
1	stalk celery, finely sliced	1
2 cups	vegetable stock (store-bought or see recipe, page 137)	500 mL
2 tbsp	snipped fresh parsley	25 mL
¼ tsp	onion powder (optional, as tolerated)	1 mL
	Salt	
1 cup	drained canned crab meat	250 mL
½ cup	1% milk or lactose-free 1% milk	125 mL
1 tbsp	all-purpose flour	15 mL

1. Spray a medium saucepan with vegetable cooking spray and heat over high heat. Sauté potatoes, carrots and celery for 3 to 5 minutes, or until slightly softened. Add stock, parsley, onion powder (if using) and salt to taste. Reduce heat to medium-low and simmer, partially covered, for 35 minutes, until vegetables are tender.

2. In a small bowl, whisk together crab meat, milk and flour until smooth. Gradually add to pot and simmer, stirring frequently to prevent clumps, for about 10 minutes, until thickened.

> **Variation:** Add ½ cup (125 mL) deveined baby shrimp with the crab meat.

This hearty soup is a meal in itself.

Lentil Soup

6 cups	vegetable stock (store-bought or see recipe, page 137)	1.5 L
2	carrots, peeled and finely sliced	2
1	stalk celery, finely sliced	1
1 cup	dried green or brown lentils, rinsed	250 mL
2 tbsp	snipped fresh parsley	25 mL
¼ tsp	onion powder (optional, as tolerated)	1 mL
	Salt	
2 cups	finely sliced fresh spinach	500 mL

1. In a large saucepan, bring stock to a boil over high heat. Add carrots, celery, lentils, parsley, onion powder (if using) and salt to taste. Reduce heat to medium-low and simmer, partially covered, for 35 minutes, until vegetables are tender. Add spinach and simmer for 10 minutes, until spinach is wilted.

Variation: Add ¼ cup (50 mL) coarsely chopped potatoes with the carrots.

Health Tip

This wholesome soup has an interesting combination of tasty vegetables that complement the lentils. This meal-pleaser is a great source of protein, soluble fiber, iron and a variety of vitamins and additional minerals. If you have heartburn and acid reflux problems, you should enjoy this soup as a soothing choice for meals or snacks.

Russian-Style Borscht

This robust red soup is the perfect thing to come home to after a hard day's work.

Tips

Garnish with fat-free sour cream, if desired.

Caraway seeds are known to dispel gas and soothe the digestive tract.

Make ahead

Ladle into an airtight container and store in the refrigerator for up to 4 days or in the freezer for up to 3 months.

2	beets (skins on)	2
1 tsp	canola oil	5 mL
2	carrots, peeled and finely sliced	2
1½ cups	grated peeled potatoes (about 2)	375 mL
1½ cups	grated red cabbage	375 mL
4 cups	vegetable stock (store-bought or see recipe, page 137)	1 L
1 tbsp	snipped fresh parsley	15 mL
¼ tsp	caraway seeds	1 mL
	Salt	

1. In a pot of boiling water, cook beets for 1 hour, or until tender. Let cool slightly. Peel, grate and set aside.

2. Meanwhile, in a large saucepan, heat oil over medium-high heat. Sauté carrots, potatoes and cabbage for 2 to 3 minutes, or until slightly softened. Add stock, parsley, caraway seeds and salt to taste; bring to a boil. Reduce heat to medium-low and simmer, partially covered, for 25 minutes, until vegetables are tender. Add grated beets with their juices; simmer for 10 minutes, until heated through.

Variation: For a creamy soup, purée in a blender until smooth.

Finally, you can enjoy Mexican food without the heartburn!

Tip

Garnish with fat-free sour cream if desired.

Make ahead

Ladle into an airtight container and store in the refrigerator for up to 4 days or in the freezer for up to 3 months.

Mexican-Style Black Bean Soup

4 to 5	strips chicken bacon	4 to 5
1 tbsp	vegetable oil	15 mL
1	carrot, peeled and finely sliced	1
1/3 cup	finely sliced green onion (optional, as tolerated)	75 mL
1 cup	drained canned black beans, divided	250 mL
3 cups	vegetable stock (store-bought or see recipe, page 137)	750 mL
1/2 cup	drained corn kernels, thawed if frozen	125 mL
2 tbsp	snipped fresh cilantro	25 mL
1/4 tsp	ground cumin	1 mL

1. Spray a small skillet with vegetable cooking spray and heat over high heat. Sauté chicken bacon for 2 to 3 minutes, or until crispy. Crumble and set aside.

2. In a large saucepan, heat vegetable oil over medium heat. Sauté carrot and onion (if using) for 2 to 3 minutes, or until slightly softened.

3. Mash 1/2 cup (125 mL) of the black beans with a fork and add to saucepan, stirring well. Add stock, corn, the remaining 1/2 cup (125 mL) beans, cilantro and cumin; bring to a boil. Reduce heat to medium-low and simmer, partially covered, for 25 minutes, until carrots are tender. Stir in bacon and simmer for 5 minutes.

This North American favorite is usually made with pork and can be a fattening addition to your diet. Chicken bacon gives the soup a lovely smoked flavor and eliminates some of the fat.

Tip

If desired, substitute turkey bacon for the chicken bacon.

The consistency of the soup should be thick.

Make ahead

Ladle into an airtight container and store in the refrigerator for up to 4 days or in the freezer for up to 3 months.

Truly Canadian Split Pea Soup

3 to 4	strips chicken bacon	3 to 4
4 cups	chicken stock (store-bought or see recipe, page 136)	1 L
1	carrot, peeled and finely sliced	1
1 cup	dried yellow split peas	250 mL
1 tbsp	snipped fresh parsley	15 mL
	Salt	
½ cup	chopped peeled zucchini	125 mL

1. Spray a small skillet with vegetable cooking spray and heat over high heat. Sauté chicken bacon for 2 to 3 minutes, or until crispy. Crumble and set aside.

2. In a large saucepan, bring chicken stock to a boil over high heat. Add carrot, split peas, parsley and salt to taste. Reduce heat to medium-low and simmer, partially covered, for 30 minutes. Add zucchini and simmer, partially covered, for 10 minutes, until tender.

➡ Health Tip

A variation of a classic French Canadian favorite, this soup provides a lower-fat substitute for smoked bacon and adds zucchini, providing another vegetable that blends well with the yellow peas, carrots and parsley. Split pea soup is a wholesome, nutrition-rich meal choice that is a great source of protein, soluble fiber, vitamins and minerals. This soup is also well tolerated if you have acid reflux.

Asian Noodle Soup

This delicious soup is quick and easy to make.

Tips

Soak mushrooms for 2 to 3 hours, or until plump.

Rice noodles can get very long and stringy. If desired, break them in half before cooking.

1 tbsp	vegetable oil	15 mL
1 cup	snow peas, trimmed	250 mL
1/2 cup	grated peeled carrots	125 mL
1/2 cup	drained canned bamboo shoots	125 mL
1/2 cup	diced extra-firm tofu	125 mL
1/2 cup	dried Chinese mushrooms, soaked (see tip, at left)	125 mL
8 oz	frozen shrimp, thawed, peeled and deveined	250 g
4 cups	vegetable stock (store-bought or see recipe, page 137)	1 L
2 tbsp	snipped fresh cilantro	25 mL
1 tbsp	reduced-sodium soy sauce	15 mL
4 oz	rice noodles	125 g

1. In a large saucepan, heat oil over high heat. Sauté snow peas, carrots, bamboo shoots, tofu and mushrooms for 2 to 3 minutes, or until vegetables are tender. Add shrimp, stock, cilantro and soy sauce; bring to a boil. Reduce heat to medium-low and simmer, partially covered, for 10 minutes. Add rice noodles and simmer for 5 minutes, until tender. Serve immediately.

> **Variation:** Substitute egg noodles made with egg whites for the rice noodles.

Salads and Sandwiches

Waldorf Salad

The addition of fennel
makes this a unique
salad that's gentler on
the stomach than the
traditional recipe.

Tip

If you're a fan of nuts,
try chopped walnuts
instead of sunflower
seeds. Walnuts have a
lower acid content than
most nuts and may be
easier on your stomach.

12	seedless purple grapes, halved lengthwise	12
1	apple, peeled and diced	1
1 cup	coarsely chopped fennel bulb	250 mL
1 tbsp	snipped fresh parsley	15 mL
2 tsp	unsalted sunflower seeds (optional)	10 mL
2 tsp	fat-free mayonnaise	10 mL
¼ tsp	dried dillweed	1 mL
	Romaine lettuce	

1. In a medium bowl, combine grapes, apple, fennel, parsley, sunflower seeds (if using), mayonnaise and dillweed. Serve on beds of Romaine lettuce.

Creamy Coleslaw

The addition of raisins
gives a hint of sweetness
to this refreshing salad.

Tip

If you enjoy a chunkier
salad, shred the cabbage
instead of grating it.

Make ahead

Spoon into an airtight
container and store in
the refrigerator for up
to 4 days.

1	large carrot, peeled and grated	1
3 cups	grated green cabbage	750 mL
1 cup	grated red cabbage	250 mL
¼ cup	golden raisins	50 mL
3 tbsp	fat-free mayonnaise	25 mL
Pinch	poppy seeds	Pinch
	Snipped fresh parsley	
	Salt	

1. In a large bowl, combine carrot, green and red cabbage, raisins, mayonnaise, poppy seeds and parsley and salt to taste. Cover and refrigerate for at least 1 hour to allow flavors to blend.

Macaroni Salad

Serves 4 to 6

This is an easy salad, perfect for lazy summer nights.

Tips

Use tri-colored pasta to add color to your salad.

Add 1 tsp (5 mL) extra-virgin olive oil to pasta while it is cooling to prevent it from becoming gummy.

Make ahead

Spoon into an airtight container and store in the refrigerator for up to 4 days.

8 oz	bowtie pasta	250 g
4 cups	assorted frozen vegetables, steamed and cooled	1 L
3 tbsp	fat-free mayonnaise	45 mL
2 tbsp	shredded reduced-fat cheese (any kind)	25 mL
2 tbsp	snipped fresh parsley	25 mL
2 tbsp	skim milk or lactose-free skim milk	25 mL
	Salt	

1. Cook pasta according to package directions. Drain and let cool.
2. In a large bowl, combine pasta, vegetables, mayonnaise, cheese, parsley, milk and salt to taste. Cover and refrigerate for at least 1 hour to allow flavors to blend.

Summer Salad

Serves 3 to 4

Rice vinegar and canned mandarin oranges are not as acidic as regular varieties. However, eliminate these ingredients completely if you are sensitive to them.

Tip

Use 1 head of iceberg lettuce if desired in place of baby greens. More fibrous varieties of lettuce, such as romaine, may be difficult to digest.

Make ahead

Spoon into an airtight container and store in the refrigerator for up to 2 days.

3 cups	mixed baby greens	750 mL
1/2 cup	drained canned mandarin orange segments (optional, as tolerated)	125 mL
1/2 cup	thinly sliced strawberries	125 mL
2 tbsp	chopped walnuts	25 mL
1/4 cup	extra-virgin olive oil	50 mL
2 tbsp	snipped fresh parsley	25 mL
2 tbsp	rice vinegar (optional, as tolerated)	25 mL
1 tbsp	snipped fresh basil	15 mL
	Salt	

1. In a large bowl, combine baby greens, oranges (if using), strawberries and walnuts.
2. In a small bowl, whisk together oil, parsley, vinegar (if using), basil and salt to taste. Pour over baby greens and fruit mixture and toss to coat.

Visits to my future mother-in-law's are never complete without a taste of her potato salad.

If tolerated, substitute 2 tbsp (25 mL) of snipped chives for the green onions.

Make ahead

Spoon into an airtight container and store in the refrigerator for up to 4 days.

Norma's Potato Salad

5	potatoes (unpeeled)	5
3	hard-cooked egg whites, sliced	3
1/2 cup	grated peeled carrots	125 mL
3 tbsp	fat-free mayonnaise	45 mL
2 tbsp	snipped fresh parsley	25 mL
1 tbsp	snipped green onions (optional, as tolerated)	15 mL
	Salt	

1. In a large pot of boiling salted water, cook potatoes over high heat for 20 minutes, or until tender. Drain and let cool. Peel and cut into 1-inch (2.5 cm) cubes.

2. In a large bowl, combine potatoes, egg whites, carrots, mayonnaise, parsley, onions (if using) and salt to taste. Cover and refrigerate for at least 1 hour to allow flavors to blend.

This sweet-tasting salad is perfect for picnics and barbecues.

Make ahead

Spoon into an airtight container and store in the refrigerator for up to 4 days.

Moroccan-Style Carrot Salad

1 1/2 cups	grated peeled carrots	375 mL
1/3 cup	golden raisins	75 mL
2 tbsp	extra-virgin olive oil	25 mL
1 tsp	liquid honey	5 mL
1/2 tsp	ground cinnamon	2 mL
	Salt	

1. In a medium bowl, combine carrots, raisins, 1/4 cup (50 mL) water, oil, honey, cinnamon and salt to taste. Cover and refrigerate for at least 1 hour to allow flavors to blend. Serve chilled.

Tips

If tolerated, you can add 1 tsp (5 mL) freshly squeezed lemon juice. Avoid if you are highly sensitive to citrus fruit.

Cut green beans into 2-inch (5 cm) slices, if desired.

Make ahead

Spoon into an airtight container and store in the refrigerator for up to 4 days.

Potato and Green Bean Salad

3	large potatoes (unpeeled)	3
8 oz	green beans, ends trimmed	250 g
⅓ cup	extra-virgin olive oil	75 mL
3 tbsp	finely diced red bell pepper	45 mL
2 tbsp	snipped chives (optional, as tolerated)	25 mL
2 tbsp	snipped fresh dill	25 mL
½ tsp	dried marjoram	2 mL
	Snipped fresh parsley	
	Salt	

1. In a large pot of boiling salted water, cook potatoes over high heat for 20 minutes, or until tender. Drain and let cool. Peel and cut into 1-inch (2.5 cm) cubes.

2. Meanwhile, in a small pot of boiling salted water, cook green beans over medium-high heat for 10 to 15 minutes, or until tender. Drain and let cool.

3. In a large bowl, combine potatoes, beans, oil, red pepper, chives (if using), dill, marjoram and parsley and salt to taste. Cover and refrigerate for at least 1 hour to allow flavors to blend.

Health Tip

The combination of cooked vegetables with different textures and fragrant herbs provides an interesting meal accompaniment. Potatoes, sweet peppers and green beans are rich sources of potassium, soluble fiber and vitamin C. This is an interesting recipe worth trying if you have heartburn and acid reflux symptoms.

Couscous Salad

This Middle Eastern salad is typically made with a lot of oil, onions and garlic. I have eliminated or reduced these ingredients significantly to suit those with acid reflux.

Make ahead

Spoon into an airtight container and store in the refrigerator for up to 3 days.

1½ cups	vegetable stock (store-bought or see recipe, page 137)	375 mL
½ cup	couscous	125 mL
½ cup	drained canned lentils	125 mL
½ cup	grated peeled cucumber	125 mL
⅓ cup	snipped fresh cilantro	75 mL
⅓ cup	snipped fresh parsley	75 mL
¼ cup	drained canned chickpeas	50 mL
3 tbsp	extra-virgin olive oil	45 mL
¼ tsp	garlic powder (optional, as tolerated)	1 mL
	Salt	

1. In a small saucepan, bring vegetable stock to a boil over high heat. Add couscous, cover and remove from heat. Let stand for 3 to 5 minutes, or until stock is absorbed. Fluff with a fork and let cool.

2. In a large bowl, using a fork, combine couscous, lentils, cucumber, cilantro, parsley, chickpeas, olive oil, garlic powder (if using) and salt to taste. Cover and refrigerate for at least 3 hours to allow flavors to blend. Serve chilled.

Variation: Substitute bulgur for couscous if desired. After the stock boils, add bulgur and cook, covered, for 10 to 15 minutes, or until stock is absorbed.

Vegetable Spring Rolls

• Preheat barbecue to high

6	mushrooms	6
1	red bell pepper, halved and seeds removed	1
2	stalks baby bok choy, finely sliced	2
1 cup	bean sprouts	250 mL
½ cup	diced tofu	125 mL
2 tbsp	reduced-sodium soy sauce	25 mL
8	large round rice paper wraps	8

Most spring rolls are deep-fried, which can cause those with acid reflux a great amount of discomfort. These are made from rice wraps, and require nothing more than a 5-second soaking in warm water. They're easy, and tasty too!

Tip

Rice paper wraps can be found in Asian grocery stores and in the ethnic section of large supermarkets.

1. Grill mushrooms and red pepper for 6 to 8 minutes, or until mushrooms are tender and skin of pepper is blistered and brown. Let cool and slice mushrooms and pepper lengthwise.

2. Meanwhile, spray a wok or skillet with vegetable cooking spray and heat over high heat. Stir-fry bok choy, bean sprouts, tofu and soy sauce for 6 to 8 minutes, or until vegetables are tender. Let cool slightly.

3. Working with one rice paper wrap at a time, soak in warm water for 5 seconds. Gently remove and lay on a flat surface. Place 2 tbsp (25 mL) vegetable mixture on the bottom edge of each wrap and fold left and right sides over filling, making a rectangle. Starting at bottom, roll up into a cylinder to enclose filling.

> **Variation:** If rice paper wraps are not available, use small flour tortillas or pita bread.

Tempeh Salad Sandwich

The nutty taste of tempeh (fermented soy) is a real treat for vegetarians, or anyone who wants to be a little adventurous in the kitchen.

Tip

Tempeh can be found in the frozen-food or refrigerated section of most health food stores or organic grocery marts.

8 oz	tempeh, thawed if frozen	250 g
1/3 cup	minced red bell pepper	75 mL
1/4 cup	grated peeled carrot	50 mL
1/4 cup	diced peeled cucumber	50 mL
1/4 cup	snipped fresh parsley	50 mL
2 tbsp	fat-free mayonnaise	25 mL
1 tsp	snipped fresh dill	5 mL
	Salt	
6 to 8	slices whole-grain bread	6 to 8
	Light margarine for spreading	

1. In a medium pot of boiling salted water, cook tempeh over high heat for 12 to 15 minutes, or until tender. Drain and let cool. Cut into 1/2-inch (1 cm) chunks.

2. In a large bowl, combine tempeh, pepper, carrot, cucumber, parsley, mayonnaise, dill and salt to taste.

3. Spread each slice of bread with margarine. Divide tempeh mixture evenly among 3 slices of bread, spreading evenly. Top with the remaining 3 slices of bread.

This exotic dish certainly beats a plain sandwich for lunch.

Tip

Add baby spinach or mixed baby greens for extra color and nutrients.

Middle Eastern Pitas

● *Preheat barbecue to high*

2	red bell peppers, halved and seeds removed	2
½ cup	sliced zucchini	125 mL
2	8-inch (20 cm) pitas	2
½ cup	Hummus (see recipe, page 124)	125 mL
⅓ cup	snipped fresh parsley	75 mL
	Salt	

1. Grill peppers and zucchini for 6 to 8 minutes, or until skin of peppers is blistered and brown and zucchini is tender. Let cool and finely slice peppers.

2. Cut pitas in half, making 2 semicircles from each. Fill each pita pocket with an equal amount of hummus, red peppers, zucchini and parsley. Sprinkle with salt to taste. Serve immediately.

Health Tip

This easy-to-prepare pita recipe has an interesting combination of hummus, red peppers and zucchini, which come together to provide a variety of textures and flavors. Pita bread provides a source of carbohydrates and vitamins. Hummus is a source of protein and soluble fiber, along with vitamins and minerals. And the peppers and zucchini are a source of minerals and vitamins. As a bonus, these ingredients are easy to digest if you have heartburn symptoms.

Using roasted red peppers instead of tomatoes gives this North American favorite a Mediterranean flair.

Tip

To roast pepper, preheat the broiler. Cut pepper in half and remove seeds. Lay pepper skin side up on a baking sheet and broil until skin is blistered and brown. Using tongs, transfer to a bowl, cover with plastic wrap and let steam for about 15 minutes. When cool enough to handle, remove and discard skin before slicing peppers.

Grilled Cheese Sandwich

2 tsp	light margarine	10 mL
4	slices multigrain bread	4
4	fat-free processed Swiss cheese slices	4
1	roasted red bell pepper, finely sliced (see tip, at left)	1
2 tbsp	extra-virgin olive oil	25 mL

1. Spread margarine on 2 bread slices. Divide cheese and roasted red pepper between the 2 slices. Top each sandwich with another piece of bread and coat the outsides with olive oil.

2. Spray a large skillet with vegetable cooking spray and heat over medium-high heat. Grill sandwiches for 2 to 3 minutes per side, or until golden brown on both sides.

Pizza

This light and fluffy dough is well worth the effort!

Easy Pizza Dough

1 tsp	granulated sugar	5 mL
1 1/3 cups	lukewarm water, divided	325 mL
2 1/4 tsp	active dry yeast	11 mL
3 cups	all-purpose flour	750 mL
1 tbsp	canola oil	15 mL
1/2 tsp	salt	2 mL

1. In a small bowl, dissolve sugar in 1/2 cup (125 mL) of the lukewarm water. Add yeast and let stand until yeast is foamy, about 10 minutes.

2. In a large bowl, combine flour, yeast mixture, the remaining water, oil and salt. Turn out onto a lightly floured surface and knead until dough is elastic and pliable. (You may need to add a little more oil and flour as you knead.)

3. Cover with a clean towel and let rise for 1 hour, until doubled in bulk.

Health Tip

This recipe provides an easy way to prepare your own homemade pizzas, a primary source of carbohydrates. The flour is a source of carbohydrates and vitamins. The addition of a touch of sugar, oil, and salt, along with the yeast, enables the chemical reaction to work in preparing a soft, flavorful dough.

Grilled Veggie Pizza

Now you can enjoy pizza without the acidity of tomato sauce.

Tips

Use floured fingers to spread the pizza dough into the pan. It will prevent the dough from sticking to your hands.

Store-bought pizza dough can be used to save time. Look for it in most grocery chains or bakeries.

- *Preheat barbecue to high*
- *Preheat oven to 375°F (190°C)*
- *12-inch (30 cm) pizza pan, lightly greased*

1	red bell pepper, halved and seeds removed	1
1	yellow bell pepper, halved and seeds removed	1
1	small zucchini, cut in thin rounds	1
1	recipe Easy Pizza Dough (opposite)	1
3 tbsp	olive oil	45 mL
1 tbsp	dried oregano	15 mL
1 tbsp	dried parsley	15 mL
1 tbsp	dried basil	15 mL
	Salt	
5	canned artichoke hearts, drained	5
4 to 5	large mushrooms, stems removed, sliced	4 to 5

1. Grill red and yellow peppers and zucchini for about 8 to 10 minutes or until skin of peppers is blistered and brown and zucchini is tender. Let cool and slice peppers in long strips.

2. On a lightly floured surface, roll out pizza dough and press into prepared pan. Brush with olive oil and sprinkle with oregano, parsley and basil. Spread peppers, zucchini, artichoke hearts and mushrooms evenly over dough and sprinkle with salt to taste.

3. Bake in preheated oven for 25 minutes, or until pizza has started to brown.

Potato Pizza

I was a picky eater growing up, but potato pizza, created by my cousin Rose Rende, was something even I couldn't pass up. This is an adaptation of her fabulous recipe.

Tips

Avoid store-bought pesto sauce, as it tends to be full of garlic and olive oil.

Be sure to spread oil right to the edges of the dough, or it will dry out during cooking.

- *Preheat oven to 375°F (190°C)*
- *12-inch (30 cm) pizza pan, lightly greased*

3	potatoes, peeled	3
1	recipe Easy Pizza Dough (page 162)	1
2 tbsp	olive or canola oil	25 mL
1/2 cup	Pesto Sauce (see recipe, page 187)	125 mL
1 cup	shredded part-skim mozzarella cheese	250 mL
	Salt	

1. In a saucepan, cover potatoes with cold water. Bring to a boil over high heat. Reduce heat and boil gently until potatoes are slightly tender, about 10 minutes. Drain and let cool slightly. Cut into thin slices and set aside.

2. On a lightly floured surface, roll out pizza dough and press into prepared pan. Spread oil and pesto sauce evenly over dough. Top with potatoes, overlapping slightly, and cheese. Sprinkle with salt to taste.

3. Bake in preheated oven for 25 minutes, or until cheese has melted and pizza has started to brown.

Health Tip

What an interesting variation of the classic pizza! The addition of potatoes provides a nutrient-rich vegetable, and the use of pesto sauce provides a tasty alternative to tomato sauce. Grated cheese provides a key flavor and texture, as well as an important source of calcium. This pizza is a source of soluble fiber, as well as vitamins and minerals.

People with acid reflux can enjoy this wonderfully green pizza without worrying about the acidity of tomatoes.

Swiss Chard Pizza Roll

- *Preheat oven to 400°F (200°C)*
- *Baking sheet, lightly greased*

1	large bunch Swiss chard, ends trimmed (about 1 lb/500 g)	1
3 tbsp	extra-virgin olive oil, divided	45 mL
2 tbsp	sliced green onions (optional, as tolerated)	25 mL
¼ tsp	garlic powder (optional, as tolerated)	1 mL
	Salt	
1	recipe Easy Pizza Dough (page 162)	1
¼ cup	shredded part-skim mozzarella cheese	50 mL

1. In a large pot, cover Swiss chard with salted water; bring to a boil over high heat. Cook for 8 to 10 minutes, or until tender. Drain and let cool slightly. Finely chop and set aside.

2. In a large skillet, heat 1 tbsp (15 mL) of the oil over medium-high heat. Cook Swiss chard, green onions, garlic powder (if using) and salt to taste, stirring, for 2 to 3 minutes, or until onions are slightly softened. Set aside.

3. On a lightly floured surface, roll out pizza dough into a rectangle. Brush with 1 tbsp (15 mL) of the olive oil. Spread Swiss chard mixture evenly over dough and sprinkle with cheese.

4. Beginning with the long edge closest to you, roll up dough jelly-roll style, tucking sides in. Place seam side down on prepared baking sheet and brush with the remaining 1 tbsp (15 mL) oil.

5. Bake in preheated oven for 25 minutes, or until browned. Cut into slices and serve.

This light pizza is not only high in protein, it's quick and easy too!

Tuna Pizza Melt

- *Preheat oven to 350°F (180°C)*
- *Baking sheet, lightly greased*

2	8-inch (20 cm) round pitas	2
1	can (6 oz/170 g) flaked tuna, drained	1
1 tbsp	dried parsley	15 mL
1 tsp	dried oregano	5 mL
1 tsp	dried basil	5 mL
¼ tsp	garlic powder (optional, as tolerated)	2 mL
	Salt	
1 tbsp	olive oil	15 mL
½ cup	shredded light Swiss cheese	125 mL

1. Spray a small skillet with vegetable cooking spray and heat over medium-high. Stir-fry tuna for 2 to 3 minutes, or until well coated with oil. Sprinkle with parsley, oregano, basil, garlic powder (if using) and salt to taste.

2. Spread oil evenly over pita slices and spread with tuna mixture. Place on prepared baking sheet and sprinkle with cheese.

3. Bake in preheated oven for 5 to 7 minutes, or until cheese has melted.

Variation: Substitute canned shrimp or salmon for the tuna.

Meat and Fish

Serves 2

For those who are highly sensitive to citrus fruit, this is a nice alternative to orange chicken.

Mango Chicken

- *Preheat oven to 375°F (190°C)*
- *11- by 7-inch (2 L) baking dish, ungreased*

2	boneless skinless chicken breasts	2
Pinch	ground ginger	Pinch
	Salt	
5	canned mango slices, cut in matchsticks	5
1/4 cup	canned mango liquid	50 mL
	Snipped fresh cilantro	

1. Place chicken breasts in baking dish and sprinkle with ginger and salt to taste. Cover with mango slices, mango liquid and cilantro to taste.

2. Bake in preheated oven for 30 to 40 minutes, or until chicken reaches an internal temperature of 170°F (75°C) and is no longer pink inside.

> **Variation:** If tolerated, add 1 tsp (5 mL) grated red onion.

Even the fussiest eater
will enjoy these tasty
treats.

Tip

Serve with Ranch Dipping
Sauce (see recipe, page
127) or Caribbean Fiesta
Dip (see recipe, page 125).

Baked Chicken Fingers

- *Preheat oven to 375°F (190°C)*
- *Baking sheet, lightly greased*

3	large boneless skinless chicken breasts (about 1 lb/500 g)	3
¼ cup	liquid egg whites, lightly beaten	50 mL
½ cup	seasoned dry bread crumbs	125 mL
1 tsp	olive oil (optional)	5 mL

1. Slice chicken breasts in long slices, 1 inch (2.5 cm) thick. Dip each piece in egg white, turning to coat, then dredge in bread crumbs until evenly coated. Place on prepared baking sheet and drizzle with oil, if using. Discard any excess egg white and bread crumbs.

2. Bake in preheated oven for 20 to 25 minutes, or until chicken is no longer pink inside and coating is crispy.

Health Tip

This quick-to-prepare low-fat recipe will become a favorite for the whole family. The crunchy texture of the bread crumbs provides a contrast to the soft chicken breast. The key nutrient in this recipe is protein, provided by the chicken and egg white. The bread crumbs provide carbohydrates and some of the B vitamins.

Meatballs lovers will delight in this delicious stew with a touch of European flair.

Mediterranean Meatball Stew

2	carrots, peeled and chopped	2
1	large red bell pepper, coarsely chopped	1
1	stalk celery, finely sliced	1
8	uncooked Chicken Meatballs (see recipe, opposite)	8
3 cups	chicken stock (store-bought or see recipe, page 136)	750 mL
1 tsp	minced fresh basil	5 mL
1/4 tsp	onion powder (optional, as tolerated)	1 mL
	Salt	
	Minced fresh parsley	
1 1/2 cups	chopped spinach	375 mL
1 cup	frozen diced turnip, thawed	250 mL

1. Spray a large saucepan with vegetable cooking spray and heat over medium-high heat. Sauté carrots, pepper and celery for 3 minutes, until slightly softened. Add meatballs, chicken stock, basil, onion powder (if using) and salt and parsley to taste; bring to a boil. Reduce heat to medium and simmer, partially covered, for 30 minutes. Add spinach and turnip and simmer for 15 minutes, until meatballs are no longer pink inside.

Variation: For a thicker stew, substitute 2 large potatoes, coarsely chopped, for the turnip.

Using extra-lean ground chicken rather than beef makes these meatballs lighter-tasting than the traditional recipe.

Tip

Use in Mediterranean Meatball Stew or serve with pesto sauce and pasta.

Chicken Meatballs

1	egg, beaten	1
1 lb	extra-lean ground chicken	500 g
¼ cup	seasoned dry bread crumbs	50 mL
1 tbsp	minced fresh parsley	15 mL
	Salt	
4 cups	vegetable stock (store-bought or see recipe, page 137)	1 L

1. In a large bowl, using your hands or a fork, mix together egg, chicken, bread crumbs, parsley and salt to taste. Using an ice cream scoop, form mixture into balls.

2. In a large saucepan, bring vegetable stock to a boil over medium-high heat. Add meatballs and cook for 25 to 30 minutes, or until meatballs are no longer pink inside. Drain and serve.

Health Tip

A great protein-rich entrée! The primary flavor derives from the chicken and broth, which is further highlighted by bread crumbs, parsley and a little salt. The key nutrients are protein, minerals and vitamins. This recipe is well tolerated if you have heartburn and acid reflux symptoms.

Using extra-lean ground turkey makes this lighter than the traditional English meatloaf.

Tip

If the mixture is too moist and falls apart when you're shaping it into a loaf, add more corn flakes crumbs, up to 1 cup (250 mL) total.

Turkey Meatloaf

- *Preheat oven to 350ºF (180ºC)*
- *Roasting pan, lightly greased*

1	egg, beaten	1
1	can (10 oz/284 mL) condensed vegetable soup, undiluted	1
1 lb	extra-lean ground turkey	500 g
¾ cup	corn flakes cereal crumbs (approx.)	175 mL
1 tsp	dried parsley	5 mL
	Salt	
	Mushroom Gravy (see recipe, opposite) (optional)	

1. In a large bowl, using your hands or a fork, mix together egg, vegetable soup, turkey, corn flakes crumbs, parsley and salt to taste. Shape into a 9- by 5-inch (23 by 13 cm) loaf and place in prepared roasting pan.

2. Cover with foil and bake in preheated oven for 1 hour. Remove foil and bake for 15 minutes, until meatloaf reaches an internal temperature of 175°F (80°C). Serve plain or with mushroom gravy, if desired.

> **Variation:** Substitute extra-lean ground beef for the turkey. Bake, covered, for 45 minutes. Remove foil and bake for about 10 minutes, until meatloaf reaches an internal temperature of 170°F (75°C).

This gravy is a great substitute for barbecue sauce or tomato ketchup.

Serve with mashed potatoes, turkey meatloaf or burgers.

For a chunkier gravy, coarsely chop mushrooms and use the stems along with caps.

Make ahead

Pour into an airtight container and store in the refrigerator for up to 4 days.

Mushroom Gravy

$1/2$ tsp	canola oil	2 mL
$1^1/2$ cups	minced mushroom caps	375 mL
$1^1/2$ tbsp	all-purpose flour	22 mL
$1/2$ cup	vegetable stock (store-bought or see recipe on page 137)	125 mL
Pinch	onion powder (optional, as tolerated)	Pinch
	Salt	

1. In a small saucepan, heat oil over high heat. Sauté mushrooms for 3 to 5 minutes, or until tender. Reduce heat to medium-low and stir in flour. Add stock, onion powder (if using) and salt to taste; cook, stirring, until gravy thickens, about 5 minutes.

➡ Health Tip

This is a tasty, low-fat gravy. The mushrooms provide an interesting texture that can be readily modified depending on how finely or coarsely they are chopped. This recipe is a primary source of protein from the mushrooms, along with B vitamins. If you have heartburn and acid reflux symptoms, this is a well-tolerated recipe.

Breaded Veal Cutlets

- *Preheat oven to 375°F (190°C)*
- *Baking sheet, lightly greased*

1 lb	veal scaloppine	500 g
1	egg white (or 2 tbsp/25 mL liquid egg white)	1
1/4 cup	minced fresh parsley	50 mL
	Seasoned dry bread crumbs	

1. Dip each scaloppine in egg white, turning to coat, then in parsley. Dredge in bread crumbs until evenly coated. Place on prepared baking sheet. Discard any excess egg white, parsley and crumbs.

2. Bake in preheated oven for about 20 minutes, or until veal is tender and coating is crispy.

Veal Burgers

- *Preheat barbecue to high*

1	egg, beaten	1
1 lb	extra-lean ground veal	500 g
1/4 cup	seasoned dry bread crumbs	50 mL
1 tbsp	grated peeled carrot	15 mL
1 tbsp	minced red bell pepper	15 mL
1 tbsp	grated peeled zucchini	15 mL
1 tsp	fennel seeds	5 mL
1/2 tsp	freshly grated Parmesan cheese	2 mL
	Salt	

1. In a large bowl, using your hands or a fork, mix together egg, veal, bread crumbs, carrot, red pepper, zucchini, fennel seeds, cheese and salt to taste. Form into 3-inch (7.5 cm) round patties.

2. Place patties on preheated barbecue and grill for 5 to 6 minutes per side, or until patties reach an internal temperature of 160°F (70°C) and are no longer pink inside.

Hearty Veal Stew

Veal is leaner than beef and helps cut some of the fat in this North American favorite.

Tip

Serve with warm Italian bread for dunking.

12 oz	cubed stewing veal	375 g
2	carrots, peeled and coarsely chopped	2
2	potatoes, peeled and coarsely chopped	2
1	stalk celery, coarsely chopped	1
2 cups	vegetable stock (store-bought or see recipe, page 137)	500 mL
1 tsp	dried rosemary	5 mL
	Finely chopped fresh parsley	
	Salt	
½ cup	frozen sweet peas, thawed	125 mL
½ cup	frozen French-cut green beans, thawed	125 mL
2 tbsp	cornstarch, dissolved in 2 tbsp (25 mL) water	25 mL

1. Spray a large saucepan with vegetable cooking spray and heat over medium-high heat. Sauté stewing veal, in batches, for 4 to 5 minutes, or until browned. Return veal to pan and add carrots, potatoes, celery and stock; bring to a boil. Stir in rosemary and parsley and salt to taste. Reduce heat and simmer, partially covered, for 25 minutes. Add peas and green beans and simmer for 15 minutes, until vegetables and veal are tender. Add cornstarch and simmer, stirring, until thick, about 5 minutes.

Pork tenderloin is one of the leanest cuts of pork, making it more suitable for those with acid reflux.

Serve with steamed rice and vegetables.

Pork Tenderloin with Dried Fruit

- *Preheat oven to 375°F (190°C)*
- *Shallow baking dish, lightly greased*

1 lb	pork tenderloin	500 g
1 cup	unsweetened apple juice	250 mL
1 tbsp	dried parsley	15 mL
	Salt	
½ cup	assorted dried fruit (such as prunes, apricots and papaya slices), chopped if desired	125 mL

1. Place pork tenderloin in prepared baking dish and brush with a little of the apple juice. Sprinkle with parsley and salt to taste. Add dried fruit to remaining apple juice and set aside.

2. Bake pork in preheated oven for 25 minutes. Pour juice mixture over top of meat and bake for about 10 minutes, until pork reaches an internal temperature of 160°F (70°C) and just a hint of pink remains. Transfer pork to a cutting board and let stand for 5 minutes before slicing. Spoon fruit and sauce over top.

Baked Haddock

This fish may be baked, but it still has the same tasty goodness as old-fashioned fried fish and chip dinners.

Tip

Serve with Oven-Roasted Potatoes (see recipe, page 203) and steamed vegetables for a nutritious fish and chips–style dinner.

- *Preheat oven to 350°F (180°C)*
- *11- by 7-inch (2 L) baking dish, lightly greased*

4	boneless skinless haddock fillets (each 4 oz/125 g)	4
½ cup	liquid egg whites	125 mL
½ cup	seasoned dry bread crumbs	125 mL
1 tbsp	canola oil	15 mL

1. Dip each fish fillet in egg whites, turning to coat, then dredge in bread crumbs until evenly coated. Place in prepared baking dish and drizzle with oil. Discard any excess egg whites and crumbs.

2. Cover with foil and bake in preheated oven for 15 to 20 minutes. Remove the foil and bake for 5 minutes, or until fish is opaque and flakes easily when tested with a fork and coating is crispy.

Health Tip

The combination of fish and bread crumbs provides contrasting textures. The key nutrients in this recipe are protein from fish and egg whites, along with carbohydrates from the grain family and vitamins. This recipe is well tolerated if you have heartburn and acid reflux symptoms.

The perfect summertime meal — grilled fish with juicy fresh fruit salsa.

Serve with steamed brown rice and vegetables for a balanced meal.

Grilled Halibut with Papaya Salsa

● *Preheat barbecue to medium*

4	boneless skinless halibut steaks (each 6 oz/175 g)	4
1 tbsp	olive oil	25 mL
	Salt	
	Papaya Salsa (see recipe, below)	

1. Brush halibut steaks with oil and sprinkle with salt to taste.

2. Place fish on preheated barbecue, close lid and grill for about 10 minutes per inch (2.5 cm) of thickness, turning halfway, until fish is opaque and flakes easily when tested with a fork.

3. Spoon salsa over halibut and serve.

Variation: Try red snapper instead of halibut.

This quick and easy salsa is a nice alternative to tomato salsa. Papaya, a revered digestive aid, is an added bonus.

Papaya Salsa

1 cup	drained canned diced papaya, ⅓ cup (75 mL) liquid reserved	250 mL
½ cup	diced drained canned mandarin oranges, (optional, as tolerated)	125 mL
2 tbsp	snipped fresh cilantro	25 mL
1 tbsp	liquid honey	15 mL
	Salt	

1. In a medium bowl, combine papaya, reserved papaya liquid, oranges (if using), cilantro, honey and salt to taste. Serve immediately.

Variation: Add ½ cup (125 mL) chopped mango, if desired.

Taste of the Orient Salmon

Who could resist the temptation of succulent salmon combined with a delicate, Asian-inflected sauce?

- *Preheat oven to 350°F (180°C)*
- *13- by 9-inch (3 L) baking dish, lightly greased*

2	salmon steaks (about 1 lb/500 g total)	2
	Salt	
1	piece (1 inch/2.5 cm) gingerroot, peeled and minced	1
¼ cup	reduced-sodium soy sauce	50 mL
1 tsp	sesame oil	5 mL
1 tsp	liquid honey	5 mL
1 tbsp	coarsely chopped green onions (optional, as tolerated)	15 mL
	Romaine lettuce	
2 tbsp	snipped fresh cilantro	25 mL

1. Rinse salmon steaks, sprinkle with salt to taste and place in prepared baking dish. Add 2 tbsp (25 mL) water to prevent salmon from sticking to the dish.

2. In a small bowl, whisk together ginger, soy sauce, oil and honey. Pour over salmon.

3. Cover with foil and bake in preheated oven for 20 minutes. Remove foil, sprinkle with green onions (if using) and baste salmon with soy sauce mixture from the bottom of the dish. Recover and bake for 5 to 10 minutes, or until fish is opaque and flakes easily when tested with a fork.

4. Place salmon on beds of romaine lettuce and garnish with cilantro.

Impress your guests with this unique and tantalizing dish.

Tip

Use less artichoke dressing, if desired.

Stuffed Sole Fillets

- **Preheat oven to 350°F (180°C)**
- **8-cup (2 L) casserole dish, lightly greased**

4	boneless skinless sole fillets	4
2 tbsp	extra-virgin olive oil, divided	25 mL
	Salt	
½ cup	Artichoke Dressing (see recipe, below), divided	125 mL
2 tbsp	seasoned dry bread crumbs	25 mL

1. Rinse sole fillets and pat dry. Drizzle each fillet with 1 tsp (5 mL) oil and sprinkle with salt to taste.

2. Spoon 1 tsp (5 mL) artichoke dressing and 1 tsp (5 mL) bread crumbs in the center of each fillet. Begin rolling fillets from one narrow end, using your fingers to keep filling in place. Poke toothpicks through each fillet to secure. Arrange in prepared casserole dish and cover with remaining artichoke dressing.

3. Cover and bake in preheated oven for 15 minutes. Uncover and bake for 5 minutes, or until fish is opaque and flakes easily when tested with a fork.

Makes 1 cup (250 mL)

Artichokes aid digestion, making them a must-have menu addition for those with acid reflux.

Tips

Choose artichoke hearts canned in water rather than oil.

If better tolerated, use ¼ tsp (1 mL) garlic powder instead of fresh garlic or omit entirely.

For a thinner sauce, increase the amount of stock by ⅓ cup (75 mL).

Artichoke Dressing

1	can (14 oz/398 mL) artichoke hearts, drained and finely sliced	1
½ cup	vegetable stock (store-bought or see recipe, page 137)	125 mL
2 tbsp	snipped fresh parsley	25 mL
2 tbsp	extra-virgin olive oil	25 mL
¼ tsp	minced garlic (optional, as tolerated)	1 mL
	Snipped fresh basil	
	Salt	

1. In a blender, blend artichokes, stock, parsley, oil, garlic (if using) and basil and salt to taste until smooth.

The surprise is how something so easy could be so good! Serve alone with your favorite dressing, or with hamburger buns as a tuna burger.

Tuna Surprise Patties

- *Preheat oven to 375°F (190°C)*
- *Baking sheet, lightly greased*

2	cans (each 6 oz/170 g) flaked tuna, drained	2
¼ cup	grated peeled carrots	50 mL
¼ cup	minced celery	50 mL
2 tbsp	fat-free mayonnaise	25 mL
1 tbsp	snipped fresh parsley	15 mL
Pinch	garlic powder (optional, as tolerated)	Pinch
	Salt	
½ cup	corn flakes cereal crumbs	125 mL

1. In a large bowl, combine tuna, carrots, celery, mayonnaise, parsley, garlic powder (if using) and salt to taste. Form into 3-inch (7.5 cm) round patties and dredge in corn flakes crumbs until evenly coated. Place on prepared baking sheet.

3. Cover with foil and bake in preheated oven for 12 minutes. Remove foil and bake for 5 to 7 minutes, or until a knife inserted in the center comes out clean.

Variation: Substitute canned salmon for the tuna.

➡ Health Tip

This easy-to-prepare entrée is low in fat but very flavorful. This recipe is full of minerals and vitamins. The combination of canned fish, vegetables, crispy corn flakes, herbs and seasonings is a real taste-pleaser. The primary nutrients are protein contributed by the fish and carbohydrates from the cereal and vegetables. If you have heartburn and acid reflux symptoms, this is a well-tolerated recipe.

Grilled Tuna Steaks with Fennel Sauce

● *Preheat barbecue to medium*

4	tuna steaks (each 6 oz/175 g)	4
1 tbsp	extra-virgin olive oil	15 mL
	Salt	
	Fennel Sauce (see recipe, below)	

1. Brush tuna steaks with oil and sprinkle with salt to taste.

2. Place fish on preheated barbecue, close lid and grill for about 10 minutes per inch (2.5 cm) of thickness, turning once, until fish is opaque and flakes easily when tested with a fork.

3. Spoon fennel sauce over tuna steaks and serve.

Fennel Sauce

2 tsp	light margarine	10 mL
1/2 cup	minced fennel bulb	125 mL
3/4 cup	1% milk or lactose-free 1% milk	175 mL
1/3 cup	warm water	75 mL
1 1/2 tbsp	all-purpose flour	22 mL
1 tbsp	snipped fresh parsley	15 mL
	Salt	

1. In a small saucepan, melt margarine over medium-high heat. Sauté fennel for 7 to 8 minutes, or until tender.

2. In a small bowl, whisk together milk, water, flour, parsley and salt to taste. Pour over fennel. Reduce heat to low and cook, stirring constantly, for 2 to 3 minutes, or until thickened.

Pasta and Rice Dishes

An excellent example of how pasta can taste good without tomato sauce!

Pasta with Peas

2½ cups	chicken stock (store-bought or see recipe, page 136)	625 mL
1	clove garlic	1
3 cups	thawed frozen sweet peas	750 mL
1 tsp	minced fresh basil	5 mL
	Minced fresh parsley	
12 oz	pasta (any kind)	375 g

1. In a large saucepan, bring stock to a boil over medium heat. Add garlic, peas, basil and parsley to taste, and simmer, partially covered, for 20 minutes, until peas are tender and liquid is slightly reduced. Discard garlic clove.

2. Meanwhile, in a large pot of boiling salted water, cook pasta according to package directions.

3. Drain pasta and combine with pea mixture.

> **Variation:** Substitute 4 cups (1 L) frozen French-style green beans for the peas.

Alfredo sauces can be very rich and fattening. I've used light margarine and light dairy products to cut some of the fat in this recipe.

Tip

Use drained canned crab, if desired in place of imitation crab.

Taste of the Ocean Pasta

1 tsp	light margarine	5 mL
¾ cup	1% milk or lactose-free 1% milk	175 mL
½ cup	shredded part-skim mozzarella cheese	125 mL
1½ tbsp	all-purpose flour	22 mL
6 oz	imitation crab meat, finely sliced	175 g
1 cup	grated zucchini (unpeeled)	250 mL
½ cup	grated peeled carrots	125 mL
8 oz	linguine	250 g

1. In a small saucepan, melt margarine over low heat. Add milk, mozzarella, ½ cup water and flour; cook, stirring frequently to prevent lumps, for 2 to 3 minutes, or until thickened. Set aside.

2. Spray a large saucepan with vegetable cooking spray and heat over medium-low heat. Sauté crab meat, zucchini and carrots for 10 minutes, until veggies are tender. Add 2½ cups (625 mL) water and cheese mixture and combine.

3. Meanwhile, in a large pot of boiling salted water, cook linguine according to package directions.

4. Drain pasta and combine with cheese-vegetable sauce.

The union of pesto with artichokes is a match made in heaven for people with acid reflux. Artichokes are known to boost digestion, while pesto is chock full of basil, an appetite stimulant and digestive aid.

Grilled Chicken with Pesto

• *Preheat barbecue to medium*

2	boneless skinless chicken breasts	2
1	can (10 oz/284 mL) mushroom pieces, drained	250 mL
1 cup	chopped spinach	250 mL
½ cup	frozen peas, thawed	125 mL
¼ cup	finely sliced drained artichoke hearts	50 mL
¾ cup	Pesto Sauce (see recipe, opposite)	175 mL
8 oz	spaghetti or linguini	250 g
	Salt	

1. Place chicken breasts on preheated barbecue, close lid and grill for 6 to 8 minutes on each side, until chicken reaches an internal temperature of 170°F (75°C) and is no longer pink inside. Slice into long strips, 1 inch (2.5 cm) thick. Set aside.

2. Spray a large saucepan with vegetable cooking spray and heat over medium heat. Sauté mushrooms, spinach, peas and artichoke hearts for 10 minutes, until slightly softened. Add chicken, pesto sauce, ¼ cup (50 mL) water and salt to taste; cook, partially covered, for 5 minutes, until heated through.

3. Meanwhile, in a large pot of boiling salted water, cook spaghetti according to package directions.

4. Drain pasta and combine with vegetable-chicken mixture.

This is a nice light substitute for tomato sauce.

Tips

If you are highly sensitive to fresh garlic, substitute ¼ tsp (1 mL) garlic powder or omit garlic entirely.

If pine nuts are not available, try chopped walnuts.

Make ahead

Spoon into an airtight container and store in the refrigerator for up to 4 days.

Pesto Sauce

½	clove garlic (see tip, at left)	
3 cups	lightly packed fresh basil	
⅓ cup	pine nuts (optional)	
3 tbsp	snipped fresh parsley	.. mL
1 tbsp	olive oil	15 mL

1. In a blender or food processor, process garlic, basil, pine nuts (if using), ¼ cup (50 mL) water, parsley and olive oil until smooth.

➡ Health Tip

This is a flavorful, herb-rich, low-fat sauce that is a great complement to many entrées. Garlic provides a rich contrast to the fragrant herbs, while pine nuts will modify the texture and further contribute to an aroma of the forest. This sauce provides some key vitamins, but is not a source of acid, making it easy to tolerate if you have heartburn.

 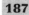

Baked Macaroni and Cheese

This requires a little more work than boxed macaroni and cheese, but it's well worth the effort!

Tip

Use all mozzarella cheese, if desired.

- *Preheat oven to 350°F (180°C)*
- *13- by 9-inch (3 L) casserole dish, lightly greased*

8 oz	elbow macaroni	250 g
1½ tbsp	all-purpose flour	22 mL
1 cup	1% milk or lactose-free 1% milk	250 mL
1 cup	shredded part-skim mozzarella cheese	250 mL
½ cup	shredded light Cheddar cheese, divided	125 mL
4 cups	frozen mixed vegetables, steamed	1 L
1 tbsp	dried parsley	15 mL
	Salt	

1. In a large pot of boiling salted water, cook macaroni for 8 to 10 minutes, until almost tender. Drain and pour into prepared casserole dish.

2. Meanwhile, spray a large skillet with vegetable cooking spray and heat over medium-low heat. Cook flour and milk, whisking, for 2 to 3 minutes, or until thickened and smooth. Gradually stir in mozzarella and ¼ cup (50 mL) of the Cheddar. Cook, stirring, until solid for 2 to 3 minutes, until thickened.

3. Combine steamed vegetables with cheese sauce, parsley and salt to taste; pour over pasta, mixing thoroughly. Sprinkle with the remaining ¼ cup (50 mL) Cheddar.

4. Cover and bake in preheated oven for 35 to 40 minutes, or until cheese has melted.

Nonna's Gnocchi

Nonna's visits were never complete until she made a dish of her delicious gnocchi. To reduce heartburn, serve with pesto rather than tomato sauce.

3	large Yukon Gold potatoes, peeled (about 1¼ lbs/625 g)	3
1	egg	1
1½ cups	all-purpose flour (approx.)	375 mL
	Salt	

Tips

Do not overcook, or gnocchi will be gummy and sticky. Remove from water as soon as they rise to the top.

Older potatoes, from storage, seem to make the best gnocchi. Avoid freshly picked ones if possible.

Make ahead

Prepare through Step 3, freeze gnocchi on baking sheets until solid, then transfer to airtight containers. Store in the freezer for up to 4 months. When cooking from frozen, increase cooking time by 1 to 2 minutes.

1. Bring a large pot of salted water to a boil and cook potatoes for 20 to 25 minutes, until tender. Drain well.

2. On a large cutting board, mash potatoes with a potato masher or a fork until smooth. Break egg into the center of the potato mixture. Gradually add flour, ½ cup (125 mL) at a time, and salt to taste; mix well with floured hands. Knead for about 5 minutes, until a pliable dough forms, adding more flour if mixture is gooey.

3. With floured hands, roll portions of dough into long cylindrical shapes about the width of your thumb. Cut into 1 inch (2.5 cm) pieces. Press your fingertip into each piece and curve into the shape of a shell. Place on a floured baking sheet while preparing remaining gnocchi.

4. In batches, drop gnocchi in a large pot of boiling water and cook for 2 to 3 minutes, or until they rise to the surface. Lift from water with a strainer or slotted spoon and transfer to a heated dish. Repeat with remaining gnocchi.

➡ Health Tip

This entrée is an easy-to-prepare meal that can be combined with the fragrant flavors of herbs in pesto sauce. The soft texture is easy to manage by all, making it a favorite for meals and snacks. The primary nutrients are carbohydrates from the flour and potato, along with a little protein contributed by the egg, some B vitamins and potassium.

Couscous is the national grain of several North African countries. Mixing it with roasted vegetables creates a delightful combination of flavors.

Tips

An equal amount of ground coriander can be substituted for the parsley.

People with acid reflux should make sure their meals — particularly vegetables — are well cooked to ensure proper digestion. Foods that are "al dente," or partially cooked, may not be digested properly, therefore increasing the risk of heartburn.

Mediterranean Vegetable Hot Pot

- *Preheat oven to 375°F (190°C)*
- *Large roasting pan, lightly greased*

2	red bell peppers, cut in thin strips	2
2	carrots, peeled and cut in thin strips	2
1	large zucchini, peeled and cut in thick rounds	1
1 cup	coarsely chopped fennel bulb	250 mL
3 tbsp	extra-virgin olive oil	45 mL
1 tbsp	dried parsley	15 mL
	Salt	
2 cups	vegetable stock (store-bought or see recipe, page 137)	500 mL
1 cup	couscous	250 mL

1. In prepared roasting pan, arrange peppers, carrots, zucchini and fennel in a single layer. Drizzle with oil and sprinkle with parsley and salt to taste.

2. Cover with foil and bake in preheated oven for 30 minutes. Remove foil and bake for 15 minutes, until vegetables are tender.

3. Ten minutes before vegetables are ready, in a medium saucepan, bring vegetable stock to a boil over medium heat. Add couscous, cover and remove from heat. Let stand for 5 minutes, or until stock is absorbed. Fluff couscous with a fork. Serve vegetables over couscous.

This dish is packed with acid reflux–friendly ingredients. India's traditional Ayurvedic healers use cilantro to treat a variety of digestive complaints.

Tips

If you don't like your noodles too long, break them in half before boiling.

To boost the flavor in this stir-fry, increase the sesame oil to up to 1 tsp (5 mL) and substitute 1 tbsp (15 mL) minced fresh gingerroot for the ground ginger.

Asian Vegetable Stir-Fry

8 oz	rice noodles	250 g
1 tbsp	canola oil	15 mL
1 cup	shredded savoy cabbage	250 mL
1 cup	finely sliced mushrooms	250 mL
½ cup	diced extra-firm tofu	125 mL
½ cup	trimmed snow peas	125 mL
½ cup	bean sprouts	125 mL
⅓ cup	reduced-sodium soy sauce	75 mL
2 tbsp	snipped fresh cilantro	25 mL
1 tbsp	cornstarch	15 mL
1 tsp	liquid honey	5 mL
¼ tsp	sesame oil	1 mL
¼ tsp	ground ginger	1 mL

1. In a large pot of boiling salted water, cook rice noodles according to package directions. Drain and transfer to a bowl; drizzle with oil to prevent noodles from becoming too gummy and set aside.

2. Spray a large skillet or wok with vegetable cooking spray and heat over high heat. Stir-fry cabbage, mushrooms, tofu, snow peas and bean sprouts for 8 to 10 minutes, or until vegetables are tender.

3. Meanwhile, in a small saucepan, combine soy sauce, cilantro, 2 tbsp (25 mL) water, cornstarch, honey, sesame oil and ginger. Cook over low heat, stirring frequently, for 2 to 3 minutes, or until thickened.

4. Add rice noodles to skillet and combine with vegetables. Pour in soy sauce mixture and stir until well coated. Serve immediately.

This hearty dish is sure to keep you full and satisfied.

Tips

Be sure to use long-grain rice, or this dish will have the consistency of risotto.

Be sure to partially cook chicken just before completing the dish. It is not safe to partially cook meat and hold until later.

Chicken with Rice

• *Preheat barbecue to medium*

4	boneless skinless chicken breasts	4
2½ cups	chicken stock (store-bought or see recipe, page 136)	625 mL
1 cup	frozen French-cut green beans, thawed	250 mL
¾ cup	long-grain white rice	175 mL
½ cup	frozen peas, thawed	125 mL
2 tbsp	snipped fresh parsley	25 mL
1 tsp	snipped fresh basil	5 mL
¼ tsp	garlic powder (optional, as tolerated)	1 mL
	Salt	

1. Place chicken on preheated barbecue, close lid and grill for 3 minutes on each side, until partially cooked. Cut into ½-inch (1 cm) pieces and set aside.

2. In a large saucepan, bring stock to a boil over medium-high heat. Add green beans, rice, peas, parsley, basil, garlic powder (if using) and salt to taste. Reduce heat to medium and simmer, partially covered, for 10 minutes. Add chicken and cook for 15 minutes, or until rice is tender and chicken is no longer pink inside.

➡ Health Tip

This inviting meal is full of color, texture and flavor. The soft chicken breast contrasts with the textures of green beans and peas. Protein is a key nutrient in this meal, along with carbohydrates from the rice and vegetables. Minerals and vitamins are also in abundance with this entrée. If you have heartburn, you should have no problems with this meal.

This dish is a favorite in my household. It's easy to prepare, and it's a great way to encourage picky eaters to eat their green vegetables!

Tip

Soy or lactose-free cheese can be substituted for real cheese.

Baked Spinach and Rice Casserole

- *Preheat oven to 350°F (180°C)*
- *11- by 7-inch (2 L) baking dish, lightly greased*

1 tsp	olive oil	5 mL
4½ cups	coarsely chopped spinach	1.25 L
1 tbsp	minced fresh parsley	15 mL
¼ tsp	onion powder (optional, as tolerated)	1 mL
	Salt	
2 cups	chicken stock (store-bought or see recipe, page 136)	500 mL
1 cup	Arborio or other short-grain rice	250 mL
¼ cup	shredded part-skim mozzarella cheese	50 mL

1. In a large saucepan, heat oil over medium-high heat. Sauté spinach, parsley, onion powder (if using) and salt to taste for 3 minutes, until spinach is wilted.

2. In prepared casserole dish, combine spinach, stock and rice, mixing thoroughly. Sprinkle with mozzarella.

3. Cover and bake in preheated oven for 45 to 50 minutes, or until rice is tender and stock is absorbed. Cut into squares and serve.

Mushrooms are an important source of nutrients and are believed to stimulate the immune system.

Tips

To soak dried mushrooms: In a heatproof bowl, pour boiling water over mushrooms to cover. Let stand for 20 to 30 minutes, or until softened. Drain, discarding liquid (or strain liquid through a coffee filter to use in vegetable stock).

Keep a close eye on this dish. As the rice absorbs the liquid, it is important to keep stirring.

Mushrooms of the Forest Risotto

4 cups	vegetable stock (store-bought or see recipe, page 137)	1 L
1 tsp	light margarine	5 mL
3 cups	chopped fresh mushrooms	750 mL
¾ cup	Arborio or other short-grain rice	175 mL
¼ cup	dried mushrooms, soaked (see tip, at left)	50 mL
1 tbsp	minced fresh parsley	15 mL

1. In a pot, bring vegetable stock to a boil. Reduce heat and keep stock just below a simmer while making risotto.

2. In a medium saucepan, melt margarine over medium-high heat. Sauté fresh mushrooms for 5 minutes, or until tender. Reduce heat to medium-low and add rice, dried mushrooms and parsley, stirring until rice is well coated. Add ½ cup (125 mL) of the vegetable stock and simmer, adjusting heat as necessary and stirring often to make sure rice doesn't stick to the bottom and sides of the pot. When rice has absorbed most of the previous addition of liquid, add more stock, about ½ cup (125 mL) at a time. Repeat this procedure until rice is tender, stirring often. It will take approximately 35 minutes to cook. The rice should be creamy, but not soupy. Serve immediately.

Fishy Rice

Christina Vieira, one of my closest friends, introduced me to a version of this delicious tuna and rice combination at her family's cottage in Northern Ontario.

Tip

You can use brown rice, but increase the cooking time by 10 to 15 minutes.

1	large carrot, peeled and grated	1
1½ cups	coarsely chopped spinach	375 mL
1	can (6 oz/170 g) flaked water-packed tuna, drained	1
3 cups	chicken stock (store-bought or see recipe, page 136)	750 mL
1 tbsp	snipped fresh parsley	15 mL
¼ tsp	onion powder (optional, as tolerated)	1 mL
¾ cup	long-grain white rice	175 mL

1. Spray a large saucepan with vegetable cooking spray and heat over high heat. Sauté carrot and spinach for 3 minutes, until slightly softened. Add tuna, stock, parsley and onion powder (if using). Reduce heat to medium-low and simmer, partially uncovered, for 15 minutes.

2. Meanwhile, in a pot of boiling salted water, cook rice for 12 to 15 minutes, or until tender.

3. Drain rice and combine with tuna mixture. Serve immediately.

Health Tip

This low-fat meal provides a balance among flavor, texture and color. The food groups are well represented, with fish, grains, starches and vegetables complementing one another. Protein is a primary nutrient, with carbohydrates, minerals and vitamins from the rice and vegetables. The spinach is a source of naturally occurring chemicals thought to be cancer fighters. This meal should be a welcome choice if you have acid reflux symptoms.

Traditional paella is made in a wide shallow pan, but today's nonstick skillet makes a very good substitute and reduces the amount of oil needed for this dish.

Tip

Try a variety of vegetables, including bite-size pieces of broccoli, cauliflower, asparagus, green beans, bell peppers and zucchini.

Spanish Vegetable Paella

● *Preheat oven to 375°F (190°C)*

4 cups	assorted prepared vegetables (see tip, at left)	1 L
3½ cups	chicken or vegetable stock (store-bought or see recipes, pages 136 and 137)	875 mL
¼ tsp	saffron threads, crushed	1 mL
	Salt	
2 tbsp	olive oil	25 mL
1	green onion, chopped (optional)	1
¼ tsp	garlic powder (optional)	1 mL
1½ cups	Arborio or other short-grain rice	375 mL

1. In a pot of boiling, lightly salted water, cook vegetables (except peppers and zucchini) for 1 minute. Rinse under cold water to chill; drain well.

2. In the same pot, bring stock to a boil. Add saffron and salt to taste. Keep warm.

3. In a large nonstick skillet, heat oil over medium-high heat. Add green onion (if using) and garlic powder (if using); cook, stirring, for 1 minute. Add vegetables and cook, stirring often, for 4 minutes, or until lightly colored. Stir in rice and hot stock mixture. Reduce heat so rice cooks at a gentle boil; cook, uncovered, without stirring, for 10 minutes, or until most of the liquid is absorbed.

4. Cover skillet with lid or foil. (If skillet handle is not ovenproof, wrap in a double layer of foil.) Bake in preheated oven for 15 minutes, or until all liquid is absorbed and rice is tender. Remove from oven and let stand, covered, for 5 minutes before serving.

Vegetable Dishes

Baked Butternut Squash

Squash is not only easy to make, it's easy on the stomach, too.

Tip

This recipe will work for various types of squash. You may need to decrease or increase the cooking time, depending on the variety and size of the squash.

- *Preheat oven to 375°F (190°C)*
- *13- by 9-inch (3 L) baking dish*

1	large butternut squash	1
1 tsp	light margarine	5 mL
½ tsp	lightly packed brown sugar	2 mL
	Salt	
	Ground nutmeg	

1. Slice butternut squash in half lengthwise and scoop out seeds. Dab margarine in the hallowed-out section of each half. Place in baking dish and sprinkle with brown sugar and salt and nutmeg to taste.

2. Cover and bake in preheated oven for 45 to 50 minutes, or until tender.

Health Tip

Butternut squash is a winter squash that is particularly rich in potassium and vitamin A. This colorful vegetable with a mild flavor and soft texture will be well tolerated by anyone with digestive problems. Squash is a low-calorie, low-fat, low-protein vegetable that is a primary source of carbohydrates.

Chinese Cabbage Rolls

Traditional cabbage rolls are made with a fair amount of tomato sauce. These Chinese-style cabbage rolls have no tomatoes and taste just as good.

Tip

Be careful not to overstuff, or the cabbage rolls will fall apart.

Make ahead

Place in an airtight container and store in the refrigerator for up to 4 days.

- *Preheat oven to 350°F (180°C)*
- *13- by 9-inch (3 L) casserole dish, lightly greased*

12	Chinese cabbage leaves	12
1	carrot, peeled and minced	1
1	piece (1/2 inch/1 cm) gingerroot, peeled and minced	1
1/2 cup	finely sliced spinach	125 mL
1/4 cup	reduced-sodium soy sauce, divided	50 mL
1/4 tsp	onion powder (optional, as tolerated)	1 mL
1 1/3 cups	cooked white rice	325 mL
1 tbsp	canola oil	15 mL

1. Bring a large pot of salted water to a boil over high heat. Add Chinese cabbage, in batches, and blanch for 1 minute, or until wilted. Drain leaves, being careful not to tear them, and lay on a cutting board.

2. Meanwhile, in a nonstick skillet, over high heat, sauté carrot, ginger, spinach, 2 tbsp (25 mL) of the soy sauce and onion powder (if using) for 3 to 5 minutes, or until spinach is wilted. Add rice and stir to combine. Remove from heat.

3. Divide rice mixture evenly among Chinese cabbage leaves. Roll each leaf into a packet to enclose the stuffing. Place cabbage rolls seam side down in prepared casserole dish and pour in the remaining soy sauce and oil.

4. Cover and bake in preheated oven for 30 minutes, until heated through.

Be sure to have plenty of warm Italian bread for dunking!

Tips

To prepare artichokes: Wash and cut off stems. Using scissors, trim sharp ends from leaves, as well as the "choke," or the prickly top part of the artichoke. Place artichokes in a mixture of lemon juice and water after preparing to prevent discoloration. The lemon juice can be rinsed off before cooking for those who are extra sensitive to citrus fruits.

To eat artichokes, pull off leaves (or petals, as they are often called) one at a time and drag them between your teeth, eating only the thick base of the leaf. The tender leaves around the base of the artichoke can usually be eaten, as well as the base itself.

Artichoke and Potato Stew

1 tbsp	olive oil	15 mL
7	large potatoes, peeled and quartered	7
2	carrots, peeled and thinly sliced	2
¼ cup	minced onion (optional)	50 mL
12	artichokes, trimmed, chokes and stems removed (see tip, at left)	12
3 cups	chicken stock (store-bought or see recipe, page 136)	750 mL
1 tbsp	snipped fresh parsley	15 mL

1. In a large saucepan, heat oil over medium-high heat. Sauté potatoes, carrots and onion (if using) for 3 to 5 minutes, or until slightly softened. Add artichokes, stock and parsley; bring to a boil. Reduce heat and simmer, partially covered, for 35 to 45 minutes, or until vegetables are tender. (The mixture should have a soupy consistency.)

Health Tip

This vegetable combination is filled with interesting textures and flavors. It is a low-fat, low-protein entrée, rich in vegetables that are a great source of potassium. This is a low-acid vegetable dish that should not be a problem if you have heartburn.

Using low-fat dairy products helps cut some of the fat in this traditionally heavy dish.

Mixed Scalloped Potatoes

- *Preheat oven to 375°F (190°C)*
- *10-cup (2.5 L) casserole dish, lightly greased*

1 tsp	light margarine	5 mL
1 cup	1% milk or lactose-free 1% milk	250 mL
2 tbsp	all-purpose flour	25 mL
2 cups	shredded light Cheddar cheese	500 mL
5	potatoes, peeled and thinly sliced	5
1	sweet potato, peeled and thinly sliced	1
	Salt	
1 tsp	dried parsley	5 mL

1. In a medium saucepan, melt margarine over medium-low heat. Add milk and flour; cook, whisking, for 2 to 3 minutes, or until smooth. Gradually add cheese and cook, stirring, for 2 to 3 minutes, or until thickened. Set aside.

2. In prepared casserole dish, arrange potatoes and sweet potato in 2 layers, spooning cheese sauce evenly between each layer and topping with cheese sauce.

3. Cover and bake in preheated oven for 45 to 60 minutes, or until potatoes are tender.

> **Variation:** Replace 1/2 cup (125 mL) of the Cheddar cheese with part-skim mozzarella cheese.

This wonderful blend of flavors is sure to delight your palate.

People with acid reflux should make sure their meals — particularly vegetables — are well cooked to ensure proper digestion. Foods that are "al dente," or partially cooked, may not be digested properly, therefore increasing the risk of heartburn.

Green Cabbage and Potato Blend

6	large potatoes, quartered	6
1	head savoy cabbage, sliced in long strips	1
1 tbsp	extra-virgin olive oil	15 mL
2 tbsp	snipped fresh parsley	25 mL
1 tsp	snipped fresh dill	5 mL
1/2 tsp	onion powder (optional, as tolerated)	2 mL
	Salt	

1. In a large pot of boiling salted water, cook potatoes and cabbage for 25 to 30 minutes, or until tender. Drain and set aside.

2. In a large saucepan, heat oil over medium-high heat. Sauté potatoes, cabbage, parsley, dill, onion powder (if using) and salt to taste, mashing potatoes with a wooden spoon as you stir, for 3 to 4 minutes, or until well blended. Serve immediately.

Variation: Boil potatoes and cabbage in vegetable stock instead of water.

Health Tip

This is another low-fat, low-protein vegetable dish that provides a good source of potassium. The herbs provide an interesting contrast to the flavors of potato and cabbage. The cabbage has naturally occurring chemicals that are thought to decrease the risk of cancer. If you have acid reflux, give it a try.

These potatoes are a delicious and healthy alternative to french fries.

Use equal amounts of dried parsley and rosemary if fresh are not available.

Oven-Roasted Potatoes

- *Preheat oven to 375°F (190°C)*
- *Roasting pan, lightly greased*

5	large red-skinned potatoes, peeled and cut in 1-inch (2.5 cm) wedges	5
3 tbsp	extra-virgin olive oil	45 mL
1 tbsp	snipped fresh parsley	15 mL
1 tsp	snipped fresh rosemary	5 mL
	Salt	

1. In prepared roasting pan, combine potatoes, oil, parsley, rosemary and salt to taste, mixing thoroughly.
2. Cover with foil and bake in preheated oven for 25 minutes. Remove foil and bake for 25 minutes, or until tender.

Quick and easy, this is a great addition to any lunch or dinner.

To julienne means to cut food into thin matchstick-sized strips.

Wash alfalfa sprouts very well before eating, as they can carry bacteria.

Stuffed Potatoes

2	large baking potatoes	2
1 cup	hummus (see recipe, page 124)	250 mL
	Salt	
1/3 cup	julienned peeled cucumber	75 mL
1/4 cup	diced red bell pepper	50 mL
2 tbsp	snipped chives	25 mL
	Alfalfa sprouts	

1. Poke holes in potatoes with a fork and microwave on High for 6 to 7 minutes, or until tender. Remove carefully and halve lengthwise. Scoop out the center of each potato, leaving 1/2-inch (1 cm) walls, and place potato flesh in a medium bowl.
2. Fluff potato flesh with a fork and mix in hummus and salt to taste. Spoon mixture evenly into potato shells. Garnish with cucumber, red pepper, chives and sprouts to taste.

Variation: Use bean sprouts instead of alfalfa sprouts.

Serves 4 to 5

Studies have shown that cabbage can help fight off a variety of cancers, heart disease and digestive problems.

Tip

This hearty side dish does call for rice vinegar, but feel free to eliminate it if you're overly sensitive to vinegar.

Red Cabbage with Apples

1 tbsp	extra-virgin olive oil	15 mL
4 cups	chopped red cabbage	1 L
2	large apples, peeled and chopped	2
2 cups	vegetable stock (store-bought or see recipe, page 137)	500 mL
1 tbsp	minced fresh dill	15 mL
1 tbsp	rice vinegar (optional, as tolerated)	15 mL
1 tsp	granulated sugar	5 mL
1 tsp	caraway seeds	5 mL
¼ tsp	garlic powder (optional, as tolerated)	1 mL
	Salt	

1. In a large saucepan, heat oil over medium heat. Sauté cabbage for 5 minutes, or until slightly softened. Add apples and stock; bring to a boil. Reduce heat to medium-low and add dill, vinegar (if using), sugar, caraway seeds, garlic powder (if using) and salt to taste. Simmer for 40 minutes, until cabbage is tender.

Serves 2 to 3

This is a great way to entice your children to eat their greens!

Tips

Substitute 10 oz (300 g) spinach if Swiss chard is unavailable.

Red or white Swiss chard may be used for this recipe.

Italian-Style Swiss Chard

1	bunch Swiss chard, ends trimmed	1
1 tsp	olive oil	5 mL
2 tbsp	chopped Vidalia onions (optional, as tolerated)	25 mL
2 tbsp	seasoned dry bread crumbs	25 mL

1. In a large pot of boiling salted water, cook Swiss chard for 8 to 10 minutes, until tender. Drain well.

2. In a large skillet, heat oil over high heat. Sauté Swiss chard and onions (if using) for 5 minutes, until onions are tender. Stir in bread crumbs and cook for 2 to 3 minutes, or until well coated.

This savory dish is a favorite in my house.

Tip

Stick to white rice, as brown rice becomes too crunchy when baked.

Make ahead

Place in an airtight container and store in the refrigerator for up to 4 days.

Stuffed Red Peppers

- *Preheat oven to 350°F (180°C)*
- *13- by 9-inch (3 L) baking pan, lightly greased*

½ cup	Arborio or other short-grain rice	125 mL
2	egg whites, beaten (or ¼ cup/50 mL liquid egg whites)	2
1	carrot, peeled and grated	1
1	stalk celery, minced	1
¼ cup	minced fresh parsley	50 mL
1 tbsp	canola oil	15 mL
3	red bell peppers, halved lengthwise, seeds and membranes removed	3
	Salt	
⅓ cup	shredded part-skim mozzarella cheese	75 mL

1. In a large pot of salted water, parboil rice for 10 to 12 minutes, or until slightly tender. Drain well and set aside.

2. In a medium bowl, combine rice, egg whites, carrot, celery, parsley and oil.

3. Place pepper halves in prepared casserole dish and sprinkle with salt. Spoon rice mixture into cavities and sprinkle with cheese.

4. Cover and bake in preheated oven for 1 hour, or until peppers are tender.

Spinach with Raisins

Liven up your greens with the sweet taste of raisins and the rich taste of pine nuts.

Tip

If pine nuts are not available, try chopped walnuts.

1 tbsp	canola oil	15 mL
6 cups	hand-torn spinach	1.5 L
¼ cup	golden raisins	50 mL
¼ cup	pine nuts (optional)	50 mL
	Salt	

1. In a large skillet, heat oil over medium-high heat. Sauté spinach for 5 minutes, or until wilted. Add raisins, pine nuts (if using) and salt to taste; cook for 5 minutes, until pine nuts are softened.

Chinese Broccoli

This tasty dish goes well with steamed rice and baked fish.

Tip

People with acid reflux should make sure their meals — particularly vegetables — are well cooked to ensure proper digestion. Foods that are "al dente," or partially cooked, may not be digested properly, therefore increasing the risk of heartburn. Cook broccoli longer if you find it difficult to digest.

1	bunch broccoli	1
1 tbsp	vegetable oil	15 mL
1 tbsp	sesame seeds	15 mL
2 tbsp	reduced-sodium soy sauce	25 mL
¼ tsp	garlic powder (optional, as tolerated)	1 mL

1. Cut broccoli crowns into florets. Peel stems and chop. In a large pot of boiling salted water, cook broccoli for 3 to 5 minutes, or until tender-crisp. Drain and set aside.

2. In a large skillet, heat oil over medium-high heat. Toast sesame seeds for 2 to 3 minutes, until fragrant and golden brown. Add broccoli, soy sauce and garlic powder (if using); cook, stirring frequently, for 3 to 5 minutes, or until flavors are blended.

This savory side dish takes less than 15 minutes to prepare.

Tip

Canned French-cut green beans can also be used; sauté for 2 minutes instead of 5 to 7.

French-Cut Green Beans with Turkey Bacon

1 tbsp	extra-virgin olive oil	15 mL
2 cups	frozen French-cut green beans, thawed	500 mL
¼ cup	finely sliced turkey bacon	50 mL
2 tbsp	snipped fresh parsley	25 mL
1 tbsp	snipped fresh basil	15 mL
¼ tsp	garlic powder (optional, as tolerated)	1 mL
	Salt	

1. In a large skillet, heat oil over medium-high heat. Sauté green beans for 5 to 7 minutes, until tender. Add turkey bacon, parsley, basil, garlic powder (if using) and salt to taste; cook for 5 minutes, until bacon is crisp.

➡ Health Tip

This is a low-fat, easy-to-prepare vegetable dish with lots of flavor. The low-fat turkey bacon provides an interesting contrast to the mild green beans, which is further enhanced by the herbs, salt and onion powder. This side dish is not a significant source of calories and should be tried by anyone with heartburn who enjoys interesting flavor combinations.

This vitamin-packed dish is a nice alternative to plain mashed potatoes.

Beta Blend

2	large carrots, peeled and coarsely chopped	2
2	turnips, peeled and coarsely chopped	2
1	sweet potato, peeled and coarsely chopped	1
1 tbsp	liquid honey	15 mL
1 tsp	light margarine	5 mL
⅓ cup	skim milk or lactose-free skim milk	75 mL

1. In a large pot of boiling salted water, cook carrots, turnips and sweet potato, partially covered, for 20 to 25 minutes, or until tender. Drain and return to pot.

2. Add honey and margarine to the pot, mashing vegetables with a potato masher. Gradually add in milk and continue mashing until smooth. Serve immediately.

> **Variation:** Substitute 1 large red-skinned potato, peeled and chopped, for the turnips.

This dish is packed with acid reflux–friendly ingredients and is sure to please your stomach.

Tip

Serve over pasta or alone as a vegetable side dish.

Herbed Zucchini

2	zucchini, peeled and chopped (about 1 lb/500g)	2
½ cup	snipped fresh basil	125 mL
1 tbsp	snipped fresh parsley	15 mL
1 tsp	fennel seeds	5 mL
	Salt	

1. Spray a large saucepan with vegetable cooking spray and heat over medium-high heat. Sauté zucchini, basil, parsley, fennel seeds and salt to taste for 10 to 15 minutes, or until tender.

> **Variation:** Add ½ cup (125 mL) finely chopped red bell pepper for color and extra nutrients.

Using light cheese helps cut some of the fat in this traditionally rich dish.

Tip

Peel trimmed ends of asparagus, as they can remain tough.

Asparagus Gratin

- *Preheat oven to 350°F (180°C)*
- *Roasting pan, lightly greased*

8 oz	asparagus, ends trimmed	250 g
1 tbsp	extra-virgin olive oil	15 mL
½ cup	shredded light Swiss cheese	125 mL
	Salt	

1. In a large pot of boiling water fitted with a vegetable steamer, steam asparagus for 5 to 7 minutes, until tender-crisp. Drain and set aside.

2. Place asparagus in prepared roasting pan and drizzle with oil. Sprinkle with cheese and salt to taste.

3. Cover with foil and bake in preheated oven for 10 to 15 minutes, or until cheese has melted.

Variations: Substitute part-skim mozzarella cheese for the Swiss cheese.

Chop up leftovers to serve with scrambled eggs.

Health Tip

You might enjoy this low-acid dish if you have acid reflux problems! This tasty vegetable side dish combines the mild flavor and texture of tender asparagus with the texture of melted cheese. The asparagus is a source of vitamin A. The cheese also contributes vitamin A, in addition to protein and calcium.

The addition of fennel seeds adds a new twist to an old favorite.

Tips

Use 1 tsp (5 mL) each dried sage and thyme if fresh are not available.

Be sure the bread is stale, as soft bread will make a soggy stuffing.

For a crunchier top, leave uncovered for the last 5 minutes of baking.

Bread Stuffing

- *Preheat oven to 375°F (190°C)*
- *9-inch (2.5 L) square baking dish, lightly greased*

3 tbsp	light margarine, divided	45 mL
2 cups	chopped celery, with leaves	500 mL
1 tbsp	minced fresh sage	15 mL
1 tbsp	minced fresh thyme	15 mL
1 tsp	fennel seeds	5 mL
½ tsp	onion powder (optional, as tolerated)	2 mL
	Salt	
10 cups	cubed (½ inch/1 cm) stale white bread (about 20 slices)	2.5 L
1 cup	chicken stock	250 mL

1. In a large skillet, melt 2 tbsp (25 mL) of the margarine over medium-high heat. Cook celery, sage, thyme, fennel seeds, onion powder (if using) and salt to taste, stirring, for 7 to 8 minutes, or until celery is tender.

2. In a large bowl, combine celery mixture and bread cubes. Spoon into prepared baking dish and mix in stock. Dot with the remaining 1 tbsp (15 mL) of margarine.

3. Cover and bake in preheated oven for 45 to 60 minutes, or until a tester inserted in the center comes out clean.

Desserts

The late Doris Kirby was known for her superb baking. This delightful bread is adapted from her yummy recipe.

Tip

Try adding unsweetened coconut, if desired.

Doris's Carrot Bread

- *Preheat oven to 350°F (180°C)*
- *9- by 5-inch (2 L) loaf pan, lightly greased*

½ cup	granulated sugar	125 mL
1 tsp	baking soda	5 mL
1½ cups	all-purpose flour	375 mL
3	eggs, beaten	3
2 cups	grated peeled carrots	500 mL
½ cup	chopped walnuts	125 mL
½ cup	golden raisins	125 mL
¼ cup	canola oil	50 mL
1 tsp	vanilla	5 mL
½ tsp	ground cinnamon	2 mL
¼ tsp	salt	1 mL

1. Sift sugar and baking soda into a large bowl. Gradually fold in flour, mixing until blended. Stir in eggs, carrots, walnuts, raisins, oil, vanilla, cinnamon and salt. Pour into prepared loaf pan and smooth top.

2. Bake in preheated oven for 50 to 55 minutes, or until a tester inserted in the center comes out clean. Let cool in pan on a wire rack for about 30 minutes. Serve at room temperature.

Health Tip

This carrot bread is chock full of tasty ingredients that are a source of important nutrients. This loaf provides carbohydrates, fats and protein in healthy proportions, as well as minerals, such as iron, and vitamins, such as beta-carotene. Just imagine the aroma as this bread is baking!

Lazy Apple Crisp

This is an easier and lighter alternative to traditional apple crisp.

- *Preheat oven to 375°F (190°C)*
- *13- by 9-inch (3 L) baking dish, lightly greased*

2	large apples, peeled and thinly sliced	2
1 tsp	light margarine	5 mL
¼ cup	quick-cooking rolled oats	50 mL
1 tsp	lightly packed brown sugar	5 mL

1. Arrange apples slices in prepared baking dish in a single layer and dot with margarine. Sprinkle with oats and brown sugar.
2. Cover and bake in preheated oven for 35 minutes, or until apples are tender.

Graham Cracker Delight

This easy dessert requires no baking and tastes a little like strawberry shortcake.

Tips

Must be eaten within 24 hours of preparation, or it will become too soft and soggy.

Prepare in a plastic container, if desired, for easy storage.

- *8-inch (2 L) square dish*

1	package (3⅓ oz/100 g) fat-free instant vanilla pudding mix	1
	Low-fat graham crackers	
4	large strawberries, thinly sliced	4

1. Prepare vanilla pudding according to directions on package.
2. Arrange graham crackers evenly in square dish. Spread pudding mixture generously over crackers. Add a thin layer of strawberries. Repeat layers as desired. Chill for 2 to 3 hours, or until mixture is set.

Easy Applesauce

This homemade delight is perfect for painful acid reflux days. It's light and easy on the stomach and takes almost no time to prepare.

Make ahead

Spoon into an airtight container and store in the refrigerator for up to 4 days.

3	large apples, peeled and quartered	3
½ tsp	granulated sugar	2 mL
¼ tsp	ground cinnamon	1 mL
Pinch	ground nutmeg	Pinch

1. In a medium saucepan, bring 1 cup (250 mL) water to a boil over high heat. Add apples, sugar, cinnamon and nutmeg; reduce heat to medium and simmer, partially covered, for 30 minutes, or until apples are very soft. Let cool and mash to desired consistency.

Applesauce-Bran Muffins

Using egg whites and applesauce cuts down on the fat and oil content that commercial muffins tend to have.

- *Preheat oven to 350°F (180°C)*
- *12-cup muffin tin, ungreased*

1¼ cup	all-purpose flour	300 mL
1½ tsp	baking powder	7 mL
½ tsp	baking soda	1 mL
¼ tsp	salt	1 mL
2	egg whites (or ¼ cup/50 mL liquid egg whites)	2
1½ cups	bran flakes cereal	375 mL
¾ cup	granulated sugar	175 mL
¼ cup	golden raisins	50 mL
⅓ cup	canola oil	75 mL
¼ cup	unsweetened applesauce	50 mL

1. Sift flour, baking powder, baking soda and salt into a large bowl. Stir in egg whites, bran, sugar and raisins. Gradually add 1 cup (250 mL) water, oil and applesauce, mixing thoroughly to prevent lumps.

2. Pour into muffin cups, filling each cup ⅔ full, and bake in preheated oven for 30 to 35 minutes, or until tops spring back when lightly touched.

The egg whites in this cake make it incredibly light and fluffy. This is one dessert that shouldn't bring on the pain of heartburn.

Tip

Cakes made with egg whites will not brown as much as cakes made with whole eggs.

Just Peach

- *Preheat oven to 350°F (180°C)*
- *11- by 7-inch (2 L) baking pan,*

½ cup	granulated sugar	
½ cup	light margarine	
8	egg whites (or 1 cup/250 mL egg whites)	8
1 tsp	vanilla	5 mL
1½ cups	all-purpose flour	375 mL
1½ tsp	baking powder	7 mL
1	can (14 oz/398 mL) sliced peaches, drained	1
	Brown sugar	
	Ground cinnamon	

1. In a large bowl, using an electric mixer, cream granulated sugar and margarine. Gradually add egg whites and vanilla, beating on medium speed until smooth. Blend in flour and baking powder.

2. Spread batter in prepared baking pan. Layer peach slices side by side and press into batter. Sprinkle lightly with brown sugar and cinnamon to taste.

3. Bake in preheated oven for 40 to 45 minutes, or until golden-brown and a tester inserted in the center comes out clean.

Variation: When in season, try using 10 to 12 purple prune plums instead of the peaches. Slice in half, remove pits and place cut side up.

...out
...n cookies

...iminating egg yolk
and reducing the sugar
in this recipe makes
these tasty morsels
lighter and more
healthful than many
commercial brands of
oatmeal-raisin cookies

Make ahead

Place in an airtight
container and store at
room temperature for
up to 3 days.

Oatmeal-Raisin Cookies

- *Preheat oven to 350°F (180°C)*
- *Baking sheets, lightly greased*

1 cup	quick-cooking rolled oats	250 mL
¾ cup	all-purpose flour	175 mL
¾ cup	golden raisins	175 mL
¼ cup	granulated sugar	50 mL
¼ cup	lightly packed brown sugar	50 mL
¾ tsp	baking soda	3 mL
¾ tsp	baking powder	3 mL
2	egg whites (or ¼ cup/50 mL liquid egg whites), lightly beaten	2
½ cup	margarine, softened	125 mL
1 tsp	vanilla	5 mL

1. In a large bowl, combine oats, flour, raisins, granulated sugar, brown sugar, baking soda and baking powder. Stir in egg whites, margarine and vanilla until a soft dough forms.

2. Drop dough by rounded teaspoonfuls (5 mL), about 2 inches (5 cm) apart, on prepared baking sheets. Bake in preheated oven for 10 minutes, or until golden brown. Let cool on pan for about 30 minutes.

 Health Tip

These tasty cookies are full of pleasing flavors and important nutrients. The oatmeal and raisins provide a great source of soluble fiber. These cookies are rich in carbohydrates, with a moderate amount of fat contributing to overall energy, and filled with vitamins and minerals. You won't be able to resist them!

Jelly Salad

Light jelly powder and fat-free dairy products go a long way in making this dessert an acid reflux–friendly treat.

Be sure the strawberry jelly is *completely* set before adding raspberry jelly.

Make ahead

Place in an airtight container and store in the refrigerator for up to 3 days.

• *4-cup (1 L) jelly mold*

1	package (½ oz/15 g) light strawberry-flavored gelatin powder	1
1½ cups	thinly sliced strawberries	375 mL
1	package (½ oz/15 g) light raspberry-flavored gelatin powder	1
1 cup	light whipped topping	250 mL
4 oz	ultra-light cream cheese, softened	125 g

1. In a large bowl, combine 1 cup (250 mL) boiling water, 1 cup (250 mL) cold water and strawberry-flavored gelatin. Stir in sliced strawberries and pour into a jelly mold. Refrigerate for 2 to 3 hours, or until set.

2. In a separate bowl, combine 1 cup (250 mL) boiling water and raspberry-flavored gelatin. Let cool, then add whipped topping and cream cheese, mixing until smooth. Refrigerate until almost set, about 1 hour.

3. When strawberry jelly is set, pour raspberry jelly on top. Refrigerate until set, about 2 hours. Unmold onto serving plate.

> **Variation:** Try using light peach-flavored gelatin instead of the strawberry-flavored gelatin and substitute 1 can (14 oz/398 mL) peaches, drained and thinly sliced, for the strawberries.

Using reduced-sugar jam helps cut some of the sweetness that can cause people with acid reflux so much discomfort.

Tip

If you don't own a pastry blender, use 2 knives repeatedly in a criss-cross motion across mixture to create a crumbly consistency.

Make ahead

Place in an airtight container and store at room temperature for up to 3 days.

Jam Squares

- *Preheat oven to 350°F (180°C)*
- *8-inch (2 L) square baking dish, lightly greased*

1½ cups	all-purpose flour	375 mL
⅓ cup	margarine, softened	75 mL
¼ cup	granulated sugar	50 mL
1 tsp	baking powder	5 mL
½ tsp	vanilla	2 mL
1 cup	reduced-sugar blueberry jam	250 mL

1. In a large bowl, using a pastry blender, combine flour, margarine, sugar, baking powder and vanilla until crumbly. Press three-quarters of the batter into prepared baking dish and spread evenly with jam. Sprinkle the remaining batter on top.

2. Bake in preheated oven for 45 to 50 minutes, or until slightly browned on top. Let cool and cut into squares.

> **Variation:** Try using reduced-sugar peach or strawberry jam instead of the blueberry.

Smoothies and Juices

Sunset Smoothie

This drink not only tastes good, but the addition of papaya can help ease your digestive complaints.

4	strawberries, sliced	4
1	papaya, peeled and seeded	1
½ cup	skim milk or lactose-free skim milk	125 mL
2 tsp	liquid honey	10 mL

Tip

Chill fruit in the refrigerator for at least 1 to 2 hours before blending.

1. In a blender, blend strawberries, papaya, milk and honey until smooth. Serve immediately.

> **Variation:** Substitute ⅓ cup (75 mL) fat-free plain yogurt for the milk. Add ⅓ cup (75 mL) water to thin the mixture out, and sweeten with honey to taste.

Berry Cherry Smoothie

This refreshing drink is the perfect way to get your daily fruit requirement.

2	ice cubes	2
½ cup	blueberries	125 mL
½ cup	sliced strawberries	125 mL
¼ cup	sliced pitted cherries	50 mL
¼ cup	skim milk or lactose-free skim milk	50 mL

Tips

Chill fruit in the refrigerator for at least 1 to 2 hours before blending.

Sweeten with 1 tsp (5 mL) liquid honey, if desired.

1. In a blender, blend ice cubes, blueberries, strawberries, cherries and milk until smooth. Serve immediately.

Vegetarians are not the only ones who can benefit from adding silken tofu to their drinks. High in calcium and protein, tofu is ideal for those with lactose intolerance and those on high-protein diets.

Tips

Chill fruit in the refrigerator for at least 1 to 2 hours before blending.

Tofu can be found in the refrigerator or produce section of most major grocery stores across North America. Look for tofu processed with calcium to get the most nutrients.

Summer Scorcher Smoothie

1 cup	cubed watermelon	250 mL
¼ cup	drained silken tofu	50 mL
¼ cup	blueberries	50 mL
1½ tbsp	liquid honey	22 mL

1. In a blender, blend watermelon, tofu, blueberries, 2 tbsp (25 mL) water and honey until smooth. Serve immediately.

Health Tip

What an interesting way to combine fruits, protein and a taste of honey! This is a low-fat beverage with a little protein and lots of naturally occurring carbohydrates. This drink is a great source of phytochemicals — naturally occurring chemicals in certain fruits and vegetables that are recognized as potential cancer fighters. The blueberries and tofu combine in that role. You will enjoy this one!

There's nothing like melon to cool you off on a hot summer day.

Tip

Chill fruit in the refrigerator for at least 1 to 2 hours before blending.

Refreshing Melon Smoothie

1 cup	diced cantaloupe	250 mL
½ cup	drained silken tofu	125 mL
¼ cup	raspberries	50 mL
1 tbsp	liquid honey	15 mL

1. In a blender, blend cantaloupe, tofu, raspberries, ¼ cup (50 mL) water and honey until smooth. Serve immediately.

Variation: Substitute sliced pitted cherries for the raspberries.

Serve this fruity blend as a snack between meals or as a healthful dessert.

Tips

Chill fruit in the refrigerator for at least 1 to 2 hours before blending.

Add ¼ cup (50 mL) water if the drink is too thick for your taste.

Fruity Splash

1	ice cube	1
1	peach, quartered	1
1	apricot, cut in thin wedges	1
½ cup	blueberries	125 mL
¼ cup	skim milk or lactose-free skim milk	50 mL
	Liquid honey	

1. In a blender, blend ice cube, peach, apricot, blueberries, milk and honey to taste until smooth. Serve immediately.

Juicing is a wonderful way to get your daily allowance of fruits and vegetables. Remember to use a juice extractor, not a blender, for this drink and all of the drinks that follow.

Tip

Do not peel carrots, or you will lose valuable nutrients. Instead, run them under cool water and scrub away dirt with a vegetable brush. Trim off tops and bottoms, as bacteria tend to settle in these areas.

If you prefer cold juice, chill produce before juicing.

Vegetable Blend

3	spinach leaves	3
2	carrots	2
1	beet, peeled and quartered	1
1	apple, cored and quartered	1
	Fresh parsley	

1. Using a juice extractor, process spinach, carrots, beet, apple and parsley to taste. Serve immediately.

Variation: Try using lettuce instead of spinach.

Health Tip

This drink is chock full of antioxidant vitamins and phytochemicals. The savory flavors of spinach and beets combine well with the sweeter flavors of carrots and apple. Potassium and vitamin A carotenoids are the key micronutrients in this drink. The vegetables used, along with the apple, have all been identified as potential cancer fighters. This is an easy drink to enjoy!

Stomach-Aid Juice

4	carrots	4
1	large apple, cored and quartered	1
1	piece (3 inches/7.5 cm) fennel bulb	1

If you don't enjoy eating raw fennel, try adding it to your drinks instead. The combination of apple, carrot and fennel makes this a sweet-tasting comforting drink for people with acid reflux.

1. Using a juice extractor, process carrots, apple and fennel. Serve immediately.

Tip

Add a handful of fresh parsley, if desired.

If you prefer cold juice, chill produce before juicing.

Health Tip

This drink is soothing for those who are having flare-ups of acid reflux. The fennel, combined with apple and carrots, acts to assist in digestion. This drink is a source of phytochemicals, contributed by carrots and apple, as well as antioxidant vitamins and potassium. This drink is a taste treat as well as an asset in controlling symptoms.

Apple-Carrot-Cilantro Juice

This drink is packed with immune-boosting nutrients, perfect for under-the-weather days.

3	carrots	3
1	apple, cored and quartered	1
2	sprigs fresh cilantro	

1. Using a juice extractor, process carrots, apple and cilantro. Serve immediately.

Tip

Substitute fresh parsley for the cilantro, if desired.

If you prefer cold juice, chill produce before juicing.

Summer Splash Juice

4	strawberries	4
1	carrot	1
½ cup	cubed seeded peeled cantaloupe	125 mL

1. Using a juice extractor, process strawberries, carrot and cantaloupe. Serve immediately.

Sweet-tasting carrots go well with almost every fruit and vegetable combination.

Tips

Sweeten with liquid honey to taste, if desired.

If you prefer cold juice, chill produce before juicing.

Refreshing Fruit Blend

1	carrot	1
1	pear, cored and quartered	1
1	apple, cored and quartered	1

1. Using a juice extractor, process carrot, pear and apple. Stir in ¼ cup (50 mL) water, mixing well. Serve immediately.

Who needs lemonade? This delightful fruit and vegetable combination is perfect for a hot summer day.

Tips

The addition of water prevents the juice from being too thick.

If you prefer cold juice, chill produce before juicing.

➡ Health Tip

As the name suggests, this drink is a refreshing combination of readily available ingredients that are well tolerated. Apples and carrots provide the phytochemicals; potassium is provided by all of the ingredients; and carrots add natural beta-carotene. A juicer will enable you to create this drink in minutes.

Ginger is known to combat nausea and vomiting and ease digestive distress. Combining it with iron-rich beets and sweet-tasting apples and carrots makes for a real treat and a great comfort drink for those with acid reflux.

Tip

Cabbage juice has proven to be beneficial in the treatment of peptic ulcers.

Too much ginger can make a drink too tangy. Do not experiment with the amount used in this recipe.

If you prefer cold juice, chill produce before juicing.

Crimson Sunset Juice

2	carrots	2
1	apple, cored and quartered	1
1	piece ($\frac{1}{2}$ inch/2 cm) gingerroot	1
1	slice (1 inch/2.5 cm) savoy cabbage	1
1	beet, peeled and quartered	1
	Fresh cilantro	

1. Using a juice extractor, process carrots, apple, ginger, cabbage, beet and cilantro to taste. Serve immediately.

Health Tip

This is an amazing drink! The mild flavor of apples and beets combine with savoy cabbage and sweet carrots to create a special beverage rich in nutrients and important phytochemicals. The ginger and cilantro add a special treat to the taste buds. It's hard to believe that something so tasty can be so good for you!

Resources

American Dietetic Association
Headquarters
120 South Riverside Plaza, Suite 2000
Chicago, IL 60606-6995
Tel: 1-800-877-1600
DC Office:
1120 Connecticut Avenue NW,
Suite 480
Washington, DC 20036
Tel: 1-800-877-0877
www.eatright.org

Association des maladies gastro-intestinales fonctionnelles
90, boulevard Ste-Foy
Bureau 105
Longueuil, QC J4J 1W4
Tel: 514-990-3355
    1-877-990-3355
Email: info@amgif.gc.ca
www.amgif.qc.ca

Canadian Digestive Health Foundation (CDHF)
2902 South Sheridan Way
Oakville, ON L6J 7L6
Tel: 905-829-3949; 1-866-819-2333
Fax: 905-829-3958
Email: CDHFoffice@CDHF.ca
www.cdhf.ca

Dietitians of Canada
480 University Avenue, Suite 604
Toronto, ON M5G 1V2
Tel: 416-596-0857
Fax: 416-596-0603
www.dietitians.ca

Gastro Intestinal Research Foundation (GIRF)
70 East Lake Street, Suite 1015
Chicago, IL 60601-5907
Tel: 312-332-1350
Fax: 312-332-4757
Email: girf@girf.org
www.girf.org

Health Canada
Address Locator 0900C2
Ottawa, ON K1A 0K9
Tel: 613-957-2991
    1-866-225-0709
Fax: 613-941-5366
Email: info@hc-sc.gc.ca
www.hc-sc.gc.ca/hpfb-dgpsa/
    onpp-bppn/bmi_chart_java_e.html
www.hc-sc.gc.ca/hpfb-dgpsa/onpp-
    bppn/food_guide_rainbow_e.html
www.phac-aspc.gc.ca/pau-uap/
    paguide/intro.html
www.hc-sc.gc.ca/hpfb-dgpsa/
    onpp-bppn/healthy_living_e.html
www.hc-sc.gc.ca/hpfb-dgpsa/
    onpp-bppn/vitality_approach_e.html

International Foundation for
Functional Gastrointestinal Disorders
P.O. Box 170864
Milwaukee, WI 53217-8076
Tel: 414-964-1799
    1-888-964-2001
Fax: 414-964-7176
Email: iffgd@iffgd.org
www.iffgd.org
www.aboutgerd.org

National Institutes of Health (NIH)
U.S. Department of Health and Human
Services
National Heart, Lung, and Blood
Institute
9000 Rockville Pike
Bethesda, MD 20892
Tel: 301-496-4000
Email: NIinfo@od.nih.gov
www.nhlbisupport.com/bmi/bmicalc.htm
hin.nhlbi.nih.gov/menuplanner/
    menu.cgi
hin.nhlbi.nih.gov/menuplanner/menu.cg

**United States Department of
Agriculture (USDA)**
Email: info@mypyramid.org
www.mypyramid.gov
www.nal.usda.gov/fnic/Fpyr/
    pyramid.html
www.usda.gov/cnpp/pyramid.html
www.usda.gov/cnpp/DG2005/
    index.html
www.usda.gov/cnpp/
    dietary_guidelines.html

**United States National Institute of
Diabetes and Digestive and Kidney
Diseases**
National Digestive Diseases Information
Clearinghouse
2 Information Way
Bethesda, MD 20892-3570
Tel: 1-800-891-5389
Fax: 703-738-4929
Email: niddc@info.niddk.nih.gov
www.niddk.nih.gov

References

Allen ML, Mellow MH, Robinson MG, Orr WC. The effect of raw onions on acid reflux and reflux symptoms. Amer J Gastroenterol 1990;85(4):377–80.

Armstrong D, Marshall JK, Chiba N, et al; for the Canadian Association of Gastroenterology GERD Consensus Group. Canadian Consensus Conference on the Management of Gastroesophageal Reflux Disease in Adults — Update 2004. Can J Gastroenterol 2005;19(1):15–35.

Armstrong D, Monnikes H, Bardhan KD, Stranghellini V. The construction of a new evaluation GERD questionnaire — methods and state of the art. Digestion 2004;70(2):71–78.

Armstrong D, Veldhuyzen van Zanten SJ, Barkun AN et al. Heart-burn dominant, uninvestigated dyspepsia: a comparison of "PPI-start" and "H2-RA-start" management strategies in primary care — the CADET-HR Study. Aliment Pharmacol Ther 2005; 21(10):1189–202.

Armstrong D. Motion — All patients with GERD should be offered once in a lifetime endoscopy: arguments for the motion. Can J Gastroenterol 2002; 16(8):549–51.

Armstrong D. Review article: Gastric pH-the most relevant predictor of benefit in reflux disease? Aliment Pharmacol Ther 2004;20(Suppl 5):19–26.

Aro P, Ronkainen J, Talley NJ, Storskrubb T, Bolling-Sternevald E, Agreus L. Body mass index and chronic unexplained gastrointestinal symptoms: An adult endoscopic population-based study. Gut 2005;54(10):1377–83.

Aro P, Ronkainen J, Storskrubb T. Valid symptom reporting at upper endoscopy in random sample of the Swedish adult general population: The Kalixanda study. Scand J Gastroenterol 2004;39(12):1289–88.

Avidan B, Sonnenberg A, Schnell TG, Sontag SJ. Walking and chewing reduce postprandial acid reflux. Aliment Pharmacol Ther 2001;15(2):151–55.

Baker LH, Lieberman D, Oehlke M. Psychological distress in patients with gastroesophageal reflux disease. Am J Gastroenterol 1995;90(10):1797–803.

Barak N, Ehrenpreis ED, Harrison JR, Sitrin, MD. Gastro-esophageal reflux disease in obesity: pathophysiological and therapeutic consideration. Obes Rev 2002;3(1):9–15.

Bardhan KD, Stanghellini V, Armstrong D, et al. International validation of ReQuest in patients with endoscopy-negative gastro-esophageal reflux disease. Aliment Pharmacol Ther 2004;20(8):891–98.

Bardhan KD. Intermittent and on-demand use of proton pump inhibitors in the management of symptomatic gastroesophageal reflux disease. Amer J Gastroenterol 2003;98(Suppl 3):S40–S48.

Barlow WJ, Orlando RC. The pathogenesis of heartburn in non-erosive reflux disease: a unifying hypothesis. Gastroenterology 2005;128(3):771–78.

Beyer PL. Medical nutrition therapy for upper gastrointestinal tract disorders. In: Krause's Food, Nutrition, & Diet Therapy. Mahan LK, Escott-Stump S (eds). 10th ed. Toronto, ON: W.B. Saunders Company, 2004.

Boeckxstaens GE, Hirsch DP, Verkleij CB, et al. Reproducibility of meal-induced transient lower esophageal sphincter relaxations in patients with gastroesophageal reflux disease. Neurogastroenterol Motil 2005;17(1): 23–28.

Boon H, Smith M. The Complete Natural Medicine Guide to the 50 Most Common Medicinal Herbs. Toronto, ON: Robert Rose, 2003.

Boyle JT. Acid secretion from birth to adulthood. J Pediatr Gastroenterol Nutr 2003;37(Suppl 1):S12–S16.

Bradley LA, Richter JE, Pulliam TJ, et al. The relationship between stress and symptoms of gastroesophageal reflux: The influence of psychological factors. Am J Gastroenterol 1993;88(1):11–19.

Brazer SR, Onken JE, Dalton CB, et al. Effect of different coffees on esophageal acid contact time and symptoms in coffee-sensitive subjects. Physiol Behav 1995;57(3):563–67.

Brown LM, Swanson CA, Gridley G, et al. Adenocarcinoma of the esophagus: role of obesity and diet. J Natl Cancer Inst 1995;87(2):104–9.

Brown NJ, Rumsey RD, Read NW. The effect of the cholecystokinin antagonist devazepide (L364718) on the ileal brake mechanism in the rat. J Pharm Pharmacol 1993;45(12):1033–36.

Brown NJ, Rumsey RD, Bogentoft C, Read NW. The effect of adrenoceptor antagonists on the ileal brake mechanism in the rat. Br J Pharmacol 1992;105(3):751–55.

Bytzer P. Goals of therapy and guidelines for treatment success in symptomatic gastroesophageal reflux disease patients. Amer J Gastroenterol 2003;98(Suppl): S31–S39.

Bytzer P. Gastroesophageal reflux disease: epidemiological challenges. Scan J Gastro 2005;40(3):247–49.

Castell DO, Richter JE (eds). The Esophagus. 4th ed. Philadelphia, PA: Lippincott, Williams and Wilkins, 2004.

Castell DO, Murray JA, Tutuian R, et al. Review article: The pathophysiology of gastro-esophageal reflux disease — esophageal manifestations. Aliment Pharmacol Ther 2004;20(Suppl 9): S14–S25.

Catarci M, Gentileschi P, Papi C, et al. Evidence-based appraisal of antireflux fundoplication. Ann Surg 2004;239(3): 325–27.

Cezard JP. Managing gastro-esophageal reflux disease in children. Digestion 2004;69(Suppl 1):3–8.

Chow WH, Blot Wj, Vaughn TL, et al. Body mass index and risk of adenocarcinomas of the esophagus and gastric cardia. J Natl Cancer Inst 1998;90(2):150–55.

Clouse RE. Psychiatric disorders in patients with esophageal disease. Med Clin North Am 1991;75(5):1081–96.

Colombo P, Mangano M, Bianchi PA, Penagini R. Effect of kcalories and fat on postprandial gastro-esophageal reflux. Scand J Gastroenterol 2002;37(1):3–5.

Compendium of Pharmaceutics and Specialties, 37th ed. Toronto, ON: Canadian Pharmacists Association, 2003.

Craig WR, Hanlon-Dearman A, Sinclair C, Taback S, Moffatt M. Metoclopromaide, thickened feedings, and positioning for gastro-esophageal reflux in children under two years. Cochrane Database Syst Rev 2004;18(4):CD003502.

Dent J, Brun J, Fendrick AM, et al; on behalf of the Genval Workshop Group. An evidence-based appraisal of reflux disease management – the Genval Workshop Report. Gut 1999;44(Suppl 4):S1–S16.

Dent J, Armstrong D, Delaney B, et al. Symptom evaluation in reflux disease: Workshop background, processes, terminology, recommendations, and discussion outputs. Gut 2004;53(Suppl 4):iv1–24.

Dent J. Roles of gastric acid and pH in the pathogenesis of gastro-esophageal reflux disease. Scand J Gastroenterol 1994;201(Suppl):55–61.

Dickerson LM, King DE. Evaluation and management of nonulcer dyspepsia. Am Fam Physician 2004;70(1):107–14.

Di Francesco V, Baggio E, Mastromauro M, et al. Obesity and gastro-esophageal acid reflux: Pathophysiological mechanisms and role of gastric bariatric surgery. Obes Surg 2004;14(8):1095–1102.

El-Serag HB, Graham DY, Satia JA, Rabeneck L. Obesity is an independent risk factor for GERD symptoms and erosive esophagitis. Am J Gastroenterol 2005;100(6):1243–50.

El-Serag HB, Satia JA, Rabeneck L. Dietary intake and the risk of gastro-esophageal reflux disease: a cross sectional study in volunteers. Gut 2005;54(1):11–17.

Fallone CA, Guyatt GH, Armstrong D, et al. Do physicians correctly assess patient symptom severity in gastro-esophageal reflux disease? Aliment Pharmacol Ther 2004;20(10):1161–69.

Fass R. Epidemiology and pathophysiology of symptomatic gastro-esophageal reflux disease. Am J Gastroenterol 2003; 98(Suppl):S2–S7.

Fass R. Gastroesophageal reflux disease revisited. Gastroenterol Clin N Amer 2002;31:S1–S10.

Feldman M, Barnett C. Relationship between the acidity and osmolality of popular beverages and reported postprandial heartburn. Gastroenterology 1995;108(1):125–31.

Flynn CA. The evaluation and treatment of adults with gastroesophageal reflux disease. J Fam Pract 2001;50(1): 57–58,61–63.

Fraser-Moodie CA, Norton B, Gornall C, et al. Weight loss has an independent beneficial effect on symptoms of gastro-esophageal reflux in patients who are overweight. Scan J Gastroenterol 1999;34(4):337–40.

Freston JW, Triadafilopoulos G. Review article: approaches to the long term management of adults with GERD-proteon pump inhibitor therapy, laproscopic fundoplication or endoscopic therapy? Aliment Pharmacol Ther 2004;19(Suppl 1):35–42.

Galmiche JP. Gastro-esophageal reflux: does it matter what you eat? Gut 1998;42(3):330–33.

Galmiche JP, Stephenson K. Treatment of gastroesophageal reflux disease in adults: An individualized approach. Dig Dis 2004;22(2):148–60.

Gambitta P, Indriolo A, Colombo P, et al. Management of patients with gastroesophageal reflux disease: a long term, follow-up study. Curr Therap Res 1998;59(5):275–87.

Gibbons TE, Gold BD. The use of proton pump inhibitors in children: A comprehensive review. Pediatr Drugs 2003;5(1):25–40.

Gold BD. Review article: epidemiology and management of gastro-esophageal reflux in children. Aliment Pharmacol Ther 2004;19(Suppl 1):22–27.

Gold BD. Outcomes of pediatric gastroesophageal reflux disease: in the first year of life, in childhood, and in adults… oh, and should we really leave Helicobacter pylori alone? J Pediatr Gastroenterol Nutr 2003;37(Suppl 1):S33–S39.

Gordon C, Kang JY, Neild PJ, Maxwell JD. The role of the hiatus hernia in gastro-esophageal reflux disease. Aliment Pharmacol Ther 2004;20(7):719–32.

Hassall E. Decisions in diagnosing and managing chronic gastro-esophageal reflux disease in children. J Pediatr 2005;146(Suppl 3):S3–S12.

Hayden CW, Bernstein CN, Hall RA, et al. Usage of supplemental alternative medicine by community-based patients with gastroesophageal reflux disease (GERD). Dig Dis Sci 2002;47(1):1–8.

Health Canada: Canada's Food Guide to Healthy Eating; Canada's Physical Activity Guide; Vitality.

Holloway RH. The anti-reflux barrier and mechanisms of gastro-esophageal reflux. Best Practice & Res Clin Gastroenterol 2000;14(5):681–99.

Holloway RH, Kocyan P, Dent J. Provocation of transient lower esophageal sphincter relaxations by meals in patients with symptomatic gastroesophageal reflux. Dig Dis Sci 1991;36(8):1034–39.

Holtmann G, Adam B, Liebregts T. Review article: The patient with gastro-esophageal reflux disease — lifestyle advice and medication. Aliment Pharmacol Ther 2004;20 (Suppl 8):24–27.

Irvine EJ. Quality of life assessment in gastro-esophageal reflux disease. Gut 2004;53(Suppl 4):iv35–39.

Jeejeebhoy KN. Heart-burning issue: gastroesophageal reflux disease. Can J Diagnosis 2003;20(1):73–80.

Johnston BT, Lewis SA, Love AH. Psychological factors in gastroesophageal reflux disease. Gut 1995;36(4):481–82.

Johnston BT, Lewis SA, Love AH. Stress, personality and social support in gastro-esophageal reflux disease. J Psychosom Res 1995;39(2):221–26.

Jones MP, Acid suppression in gastroesophaeal reflux disease: Why? How? How much and when? Pastgrad Med J 2002;78(922):465–68.

Kahrilas PJ. Diagnosis of symptomatic gastroesophaeal reflux disease. Amer J Gastroenterol 2003;98(Suppl 3):S15–S23.

Kamolz T, Granderath FA, Pointner R. Does major depression in patients with gastroesophageal reflux disease affect the outcome of laproscopic antireflux surgery? Surg Endosc 2003;17(1):55–60.

Kamolz T, Velanovich V. Psychological and emotional aspects of gastro-esophageal reflux disease. Dis Esophagus 2002;15(3):199–203.

Kamolz T, Pointner R, Velanovich V. The impact of gastroesophageal reflux disease on quality of life. Surg Endosc 2003;17(8):1193–99.

Kamolz T, Pointner R. Gastroesophgeal reflux disease: Heartburn from a psychological view. Minerva Gastroenterol Dietol 2004;50(3):261–68.

Katelaris PH. An evaluation of current GERD therapy: A summary and comparison of effectiveness, adverse effects and costs of drugs, surgery and endoscopic therapy. Best Practice & Res Clin Gastroenterol 2004;18(S):39–45.

Kendall-Reed P, Reed, S. The Complete Doctor's Stress Solution: Understanding, Treating, and Preventing Stress and Stress-Related Illnesses. Toronto, ON: Robert Rose, 2004.

Kinoshita Y. Review article: Treatment of gastro-esophageal reflux disease — lifestyle advice and medication. Aliment Pharmacol Ther 2004;20 (Suppl 8):19–23.

Kjellin A, Ramel S, Rossner S, Thor K. Gastroesophageal reflux in obese patients is not reduced by weight reduction. Scand J Gastroenterol 1996;31(11):1047–51.

Kock GH, Tack J, Sifrim D et al. The role of acid and duodenal gastroesophageal reflux in symptomatic GERD. Amer J Gastroenterol 2001;96(7):2033–40.

Lagergren J. Adenocarcinoma of oesophagus: what exactly is the size of the problem and who is at risk? Gut 2005;54(Suppl 1):i1–5.

Locke RG. Natural history of nonerosive reflux disease. Is all gastroesophaeal reflux the same? What is the evidence? Gastroenterol Clin N Amer 2002;31: S59–S66.

Lundell L. Surgery of gastroesophageal reflux disease: a competitive or complementary procedure? Dig Dis 2004;22(2):161–70.

Marteau P, Seksik P. Tolerance of probiotics and prebiotics. J Clin Gastroenterol 2004 38(6 Suppl):S67–S69.

Martini FH. The digestive system. In: Fundamentals of Anatomy and Physiology. Martini FH (ed). 6th ed. San Francisco, CA: Pearson Education, Benjamin Cummings, 2004, pp. 882–94.

Mayne ST, Navarro SA, Diet, obesity and reflux in the etiology of adenocarcinomas of the esophagus and gastric cardia in humans. J Nutr 2002 132(Suppl 11):3467S–3470S.

Mayne ST, Risch HA, Dubrow R, et al. Nutrient intake and risk of subtypes of esophageal and gastric cancer. Cancer Epidemiol Biomarkers Prev 2001; 10(10):1055–62.

Meining A, Classen M. The role of diet and lifestyle measures in the pathogenesis and treatment of gastroesophageal reflux disease. Am J Gastroenterol 2000;95(10):2692–97.

Meyer JH, Lembo A, Elashoff JD, et al. Duodenal fat intensifies the perception of heartburn. Gut; 2001:49(5):624–28.

McDonald-Haile J, Bradley LA, Bailey MA, et al. Relaxation training reduces symptom reports and acid exposure in patients with gastroesophageal reflux disease. Gastroenterology 1994;107(1): 61–69.

Mittal RK. Pathophysiology of gastroesophageal reflux: motility factors. J Gastroenterol 2003;38(Suppl 15):7–12.

Mittal RK. Do we understand how surgery prevents gastroesophageal reflux? Gastroenterology 1994;106(6): 1714–16.

Modlin I, Kidd M. GERD 2004: Issues from the past and a consensus for the future. Best Practice & Res Clin Gastroenterol 2004;18(S):55–66.

Modlin IM, Moss SF, Kidd M, Lye KD. Gastroesophageal reflux disease: then and now. J Clin Gastroenterol 2004; 38(5):390–402.

Monnikes H, Bardhan KD, Stanghelli V, et al. Evaluation of GERD symptoms during therapy. Part II. Psychometric evaluation and validation of the new questionnaire ReQuest in erosive GERD. Digestion 2004;69(4):238–44.

Moss SF, Armstrong D, Arnold R, et al. GERD 2003 – a consensus on the way ahead. Digestion 2003;67(3):111–17.

Murray L, Johnston B, Lane A, et al. Relationship between body mass and gastro-esophageal reflux symptoms: The Bristol Helicobacter Project. Int J Epidemiol 2003;32(4):645–50.

Naliboff BD, Mayer M, Fass R et al. The effect of life stress on symptoms of heartburn. Psychosom Med 2004; May–June;66(3):426–34.

Nandurkar S, Locke GR, Fett S, et al. Relationship between body mass index, diet, exercise, and gastroesophageal reflux symptoms in a community. Aliment Pharmacol Ther 2004;20(5): 497–505.

National Academy of Sciences: Dietary Reference Intakes, 2000.

Neumayer C, Ciovica R, Gadenstatter M, et al. Significant weight loss after Nissen fundoplication. Surg Endosc 2005;19: 15–20.

Nilsson M, Johnsen R, Ye W, et al. Lifestyle related risk factors in the aetiology of gastro-esophageal reflux. Gut 2004; 53(12):1730–35.

Nilsson M, Johnsen R, Ye W, et al. Prevalence of gastro-esophageal reflux symptoms and the influence of age and sex. Scan J Gastrenterol 2004;39: 1040–45.

Nilsson M, Lagergren J. The relation between body mass and gastro-oesophageal reflux. Best Practice & Res Clin Gastroenterol 2004;18(6):1117–23.

Nilsson M, Lundegardh G, Carling L, et al. Body mass and reflux esophagitis: An oestrogen-dependent association? Scand J Gastroenterol 2002;37(6):626–30.

Nilsson M, Wenner J, Larsson S, Johnsson F. Randomized clinical trial of laproscopic versus open fundoplication for gastro-esophageal reflux. Br J Surg 2004;91(5):552–59.

Ofman JJ. The economic and quality of life impact of symptomatic gastro-esophageal reflux disease. Amer J Gastroenterol 2003;98(Suppl):S8–S14.

Olden KW. The psychological aspects of noncardiac chest pain. Gastroenterol Clin North Am 2004;33(1):61–67.

O'Leary C, McCarthy J, Humphries M, et al. The prophylactic use of a proton pump inhibitor before food and alcohol. Aliment Pharmacol Ther 2003;17(5): 683–86.

Pacini F, Calabrese C, Cipolletta L. Burden of illness in Italian patients with gastroesophgeal reflux disease. Curr Med Res Opin 2005;21(4):495–502.

Palmer K. Review article: Indications for anti-reflux surgery and endoscopic anti-reflux procedures. Aliment Pharmacol Ther 2004;20(Suppl 8):32–35.

Pare P, Meyer F, Armstrong D, et al. Validation of the GSFQ, a self-administered symptom frequency questionnaire for patients with gastro-esophageal reflux disease. Can J Gastroenterol 2003;17(5):307–12.

Pehl C, Pfeiffer A, Waizenhoefer A, et al. Effect of caloric density of a meal on lower esophageal sphincter motility and gastro-esophageal reflux in healthy subjects. Aliment Pharmacol Ther 2001;15(2):233–39.

Pehl C, Waizenhoefer A, Wendl B, et al. Effect of low and high fat meals on lower esophageal sphincter motility and gastroesophgeal reflux in healthy subjects. Am J Gastroenterol 1999;94(5): 1192–96.

Penagini R. Fat and gastro-esophageal reflux disease. Eur J Gastroenterol Hepatol 2000;12(12):1343–45.

Penagini R, Mangano M, Bianchi PA. Effect of increasing the fat content but not the energy load of a meal on gastro-esophageal reflux and lower oesophgeal sphincter motor function. Gut 1998; 42(3):330–33.

Piche T, Zerbib F, Bruley des Varannes S, et al. Modulation by colonic fermentation of LES function in humans. Am J Physiol Gastrointest Liver Physiol 2000;278:G578–G584.

Piche T, des Varannes SB, Sacher-Huvelin S, et al. Colonic fermentation influences lower esophageal sphincter function in gastroesophageal reflux disease. Gastroenterology 2003; 124(4):894–902.

Picca SM, et al. Motility disorders during pregnancy. Ann Int Med 1993;119:637.

Plynn CA. The evaluation and of adults with gastroesophageal reflux disease. J Family Pract 2001;50(1):57–63.

Prasad M, Rentz AM, Revicki DA. The impact of treatment of gastroesophageal reflux disease on health-related quality of life: A literature review. Pharmaoeconomics 2003; 21(11):769–90.

Priddle M. Gastro-esophageal reflux disease (GERD), Apotex Inc, Pharmawise Newsletter, 7(2) March 2003.

Quigley, EMM. Factors that influence therapeutic outcomes in symptomatic gastroesophageal reflux disease. Amer J Gastroenterol 2003;98(Suppl 3):S24–S30.

Raiha I, Impivaara O, Seppala M, et al. Determinants of symptoms suggestive of gastroesophageal reflux disease in the elderly. Scand J Gastroenterol 1993; 28(11):1011–14.

Ramirez FC. Diagnosis and treatment of gastro-esophageal reflux disease in the elderly. Cleve Clin J Med 2000;67(10): 755–66.

Revicki DA, Wood M, Maton PN, Sorensen S. The impact of gastroesophageal reflux disease on health-related quality of life. Am J Med 1998;104(3):252–58.

Richter JE, Hewson EG, Sinclair JW, Dalton CB. Acid perfusion test and 24-hour esophageal pH monitoring with symptom index. Comparison of tests for esophageal acid sensitivity. Dig Dis Sci 1991;36(5):565–71.

Romagnuolo J. Endoscopic "antireflux" procedures: Not yet ready for prime time. Can J Gastroenterol 2004; 18(9):573–577.

Ronkainen J, Aro P, Storskrubb T, et al. High prevalence of gastroesophageal reflux symptoms and esophagitis with or without symptoms in the general adult Swedish population: a Kalixanda study report. Scan J Gastrenterol 2005; 40(3):275–85.

Ruhl CE, Everhart JE. Overweight, but not high dietary intake, increases risk of gastro-esophageal reflux disease hospitalization: the NHANES I epidemiological followup study. Ann Epidemiol 1999; 9(2):424–35.

Safadi BY. Laproscopic antireflux surgery. Minerva Chir 2004;59(5):447–59.

Salvatore S, Hauser B, Vandenplas Y. The natural course of gastro-esophageal reflux. Acta Pediatr 2004;93(8): 1063–69.

Salvatore S, Vandenplas Y. Gastro-esophageal reflux disease and motility disorders. Best Practice & Res Clin Gastroenterol 2003;17(2):163–79.

Sarani B, Scanlon J, Jackson P, Evans SR. Selection criteria among gastroenterologists and surgeons for laproscopic antirelux surgery. Surg Endosc 2002;16(1):57–63.

Shah A, Uribe J, Katz PO. Gastroesophageal reflux disease and obesity. Gastroenterol Clin North Am 2005;34(1):35–43.

Shay SS, Conwell DL, Mehindru V, Hertz B. The effect of posture on gastro-esophageal reflux event frequency and composition during fasting. Am J Gastroenterol 1996;91(1):54–60.

Spiller RC, Trotman IF, Higgins BE, et al. The ileal brake – inhibition of jejunal motility after ileal fat perfusion in man. Gut 1984;25(4):365–74.

Spiller RC, Trotman IF, Adrian TE, et al. Further characterization of the 'ileal brake' reflex in man – effect of ileal infusion of partial digests of fat, protein, and starch on jejunal motility and release of neurotensin, enteroglucagon, and peptide YY. Gut 1988;29(8):1042–51.

Spitz L, McLeod E. Gastro-esophageal reflux. Semin Pediatr Surg 2003; 12(4):237–40.

Stein MR (Ed). Gastroesophageal Reflux Disease and Airway Disease. New York, NY: Marcel Dekker, Inc., 1999.

Stenson WF. The esophagus and stomach. In: Modern Nutrition in Health and Disease, Shils, ME, Olson JA, Shike M, Ross AC (eds), 9th ed. Philadelphia, PA: Lippincott, Williams and Wilkins, 1999, pp. 1125–30.

Stranghellini V, Armstrong D, Monnikes H, Bardhan KD. Systematic review: Do we need a new gastro-esophageal reflux disease questionnaire? Aliment Pahrmacolo Ther 2004;19(5):463–79.

Talley NJ, Wiklund I. Patient reported outcomes in gastroesophageal reflux disease: an overview of available measures. Qual Life Res 2005;14(1):21–33.

Tam W, Dent J. Oesophageal disorders: future developments. Best Practice & Res Clin Gastroenterol 2002;16(6):811–33.

Terry P, Lagergren J, Ye W, et al. Antioxidants and cancers of the esophagus and gastric cardia. Int J Cancer 2000;87(5):750–54.

Terry P, Lagergren J, Wolk A, Nyren O. Reflux-inducing dietary factors and risk of adenocarcinoma of the esophagus and gastric cardia. Nutr Cancer 2000; 38(2):186–91.

Terry P, Lagergren J, Ye W, et al. Inverse association between intake of cereal fiber and risk of gastric cardia cancer. Gastroenterol 2001;120(2):387–91.

Thomson AB, Barkun AN, Armstrong D. The prevalence of clinically significant endoscopic findings in primary care patients with uninvestigated dyspepsia: the Canadian Adult Dyspepsia Empiric Treatment — Prompt Endoscopy (CADET-PE) study. Aliment Pharmcol Therapeutics 2003;17(12):1481–91.

Tougas G, Chen Y, Hwang P, Liu M, Eggleston A. Prevalence and impact of upper gastrointestinal symptoms in the Canadian population: Findings from the DIGEST study. Domestic/International Gastroenterology Surveillance Study. Am J Gastroenterol 1999;94:2845–54.

Tytgat GN. Are there unmet needs in acid suppression? Best Practice & Res Clin Gastroenterol 2004;18(S)67–72.

Tytgat GN. Review article: Treatment of mild and severe cases of GERD. Aliment Pharmacol Ther 2002;16(Suppl 4):73–78.

Van Herwaarden MA, Smout JPM. Diagnosis of reflux disease. Best Practice & Res Clin Gastroenterol 2000;14(5):759–74.

Vanderhoff BT, Tahboub RM. Proton pump inhibitors: An update. Amer Fam Physician 2002;66:273–80.

Velanovich V. The effect of chronic pain syndromes and psychoemotional disorders on symptomatic and quality-of-life outcomes of antireflux surgery. J Gastrointest Surg 2003;7(1):53–58.

Velanovich V, Karmy-Jones R. Psychiatric disorders affect outcomes of antireflux operations for gastroesophageal reflux disease. Surg Endosc 2001; 15(2):171–75.

Veldhuyzen van Zanten SJ, Bradette M, Chiba N, et al. Evidence-based recommendations for short- and long-term management of uninvestigated dyspepsia in primary care: an update of the Canadian Dyspepsia Working Group (CanDys) clinical management tool. Can J Gastroenterol 2005;19(5):285–303.

Vandenplas Y, Hassall E. Mechanisms of gastroesophageal reflux and gastroesophageal reflux disease. J Pediatr Gastroenterol Nutr 2002;35(2):119–36.

Washington N, Steele RJ, Jackson SJ, et al. Patterns of food and acid reflux in patients with low-grade oesophagitis — the role of an anti-reflux agent. Aliment Pharmcol Ther 1998;12(1):53–58.

Wiklund I, Butler-Wheelhouse P. Psychosocial factors and their role in symptomatic gastroesophageal reflux disease and functional dyspepsia. Scand J Gastroenterol Suppl 1996;220:94–100.

Wiklund I. Review of the quality of life and burden of illness in gastroesophageal reflux disease. Dig Dis 2004;22(2):108–14.

Wildi SM, Tutuian R, Castell DO. The influence of rapid food intake on postprandial reflux: studies in healthy volunteers. Am J Gastroenterol 2004;99(9):1645–51.

Wilkinson S. Clinician's Guide to Oesophageal Diseases. London, UK: Chapman & Hall Medical, 1981.

Wong WM, Lam KF, Cheng C, et al. Population-based study of noncardiac chest pain in southern Chinese: Prevalence, psychosocial factors and health care utilization. World J Gastroenterol 2004;10(5):707–12.

Wu AH, Tseng CC, Bernstein L. Hiatal hernia, reflux symptoms, body size, and risk of esophageal and gastric adenocarcinoma. Cancer 2003;98(5): 940–48.

Xing J, Chen JD. Alterations of gastrointestinal motility in obesity. Obes Res. 2004;12(11):1723–32.

Zhang ZF, Kurtz RC, Yu GP, et al. Adenocarcinoma of the esophagus and gastric cardia: the role of diet. Nutr Cancer 1997;27(3):298–309.

Glossary

Acid indigestion: an uncomfortable feeling of heartburn, fullness, and bloating, with a sour taste of acid in the throat or mouth

Acid reflux: the backing up of stomach acid into the esophagus, often but not always following meals

Acid reflux disease: when problems with acid reflux occur regularly, require medical therapy and interfere one's life

Antacid: medications that are used to neutralize hydrochloric acid from the stomach; they can be purchased over the counter without a prescription

Barrett's esophagus: changes in tissue at the lower end of the esophagus; the tissue changes might increase the risk of esophageal cancer

Diaphragm: the muscular and fibrous tissue that separates the thoracic, or chest, cavity from the abdominal cavity

Digestive enzyme: any enzyme within the digestive system that acts to facilitate the chemical breakdown of protein, fat, or carbohydrate to enable their absorption within the digestive tract

Digestive juices/secretions: a thin fluid secreted by glands within the stomach; it is made up of hydrochloric acid, some digestive enzymes, and mucus

Digestive tract: the hollow muscular tube, lined with a mucus membrane, that runs from the mouth to the anus

Dysphagia: difficulty in swallowing, often as a result of an obstruction of the esophagus or problems with muscular coordination between the mouth and the lower esophagus

Endoscopy: the use of a specialized camera to view the interior of organs and cavities within the body

Esophageal cancer: malignant tumor of the esophagus that occurs more frequently in men than in women

Esophageal erosions: small tears of the esophageal mucosal tissue that can occur in some people who have GERD

Esophagitis: an inflammatory reaction within the mucosal tissue of the esophagus

Esophagus: the muscular hollow tube that links the back of the throat to the stomach

Fundoplication: a surgical procedure to treat an incompetent LES muscle that involves creating folds of tissue using the upper part of the stomach

Gastroenterologist: a medical doctor who has specialized training to diagnose and treat people with diseases of the digestive system

Gastroesophageal reflux (GER): backup of acid from the stomach into the esophagus, which causes a burning pain in the esophagus, usually as a result of a LES muscle that is not functioning normally

Gastroesophageal reflux disease (GERD): when problems with GER occur regularly, require medical therapy and interfere one's life, the disorder is considered a disease

Gastroparesis: changes in the motility of the stomach that interfere with the normal emptying of the stomach

Gastroscopy (see Endoscopy): the use of a specialized camera to view the interior of the upper digestive system, from the mouth into the stomach, and beyond into the upper part of the small bowel

Heartburn: a painful sensation within the esophagus, felt as a burning in the chest area, behind the breastbone

Helicobacter pylori (H. pylori): a species of bacteria that is found in the mucosal tissues of the stomach; associated with gastric and peptic ulcer disease

Hiatus/hiatal hernia: movement of the upper part of the stomach through the diaphragm; it may be a cause of GERD in some people

Histamine receptor antagonists (H2-RAs or H2 blockers): a class of medications that interfere with the stimulation of cells within the stomach by histamine

Hydrochloric acid: main substance found in gastric juice; it is found in the stomach and acts to break down foods entering the digestive system

Laryngitis: an inflammatory reaction of the mucosal tissue lining the larynx; vocal cord swelling and a hoarse voice are associated with laryngitis

Lower esophageal sphincter (LES): powerful circular muscle located between the esophagus and the stomach; it controls that passage of fluids and solids from the esophagus into the stomach

Mucosal membrane/tissue: thin sheets of tissue that cover or line the interior of various organs within the body

Mucus: slippery fluid that is secreted by mucus membranes or glands

Parietal cell: cells found on the peripheral edge of glands within the stomach; they provide hydrochloric acid within the stomach

Peristaltic waves: regulated contractions that occur within the digestive system to propel food from the mouth throughout the digestive tract

Prokinetic agent: a class of medications that act to facilitate the movement of digestive content from the stomach into the small bowel

Proton pump inhibitor (PPI): medication that inhibits the secretion of gastric acid in the stomach by blocking the action of the hydrogen-potassium-ATPase enzyme at the parietal cell within the stomach

Pyloric sphincter (pylorus): a circular band of muscle that opens and closes off the opening between the stomach and the small bowel

Reflux: the backward movement of hydrochloric acid and pepsin from the stomach into the esophagus

Saliva: clear fluid produced by the salivary and mucus glands within the mouth

Sphincter muscle: a circular band of muscle that opens and closes off an opening in the body, as in opening or closing off a part of the digestive tract

Upper esophageal sphincter: powerful circular muscle located between the throat and the esophagus; it controls that passage of fluids and solids from the throat into the esophagus

Valve: within the body, valves act to prevent the backing up or refluxing of fluid that passes through them

Acknowledgments

The writing of a book such as this can only be achieved through the efforts of many. A special thanks goes to Bob Dees, our publisher, and Marian Jarkovich, Sales and Marketing Manager at Robert Rose Inc. Thanks also to Bob Hilderley, our health editor, who truly made the book "come alive," to Sue Sumeraj, our recipe editor, and to Jennifer MacKenzie, our recipe tester, all of whom have done a great job supporting and assisting us during this project. David Armstrong, MD, Division of Gastroenterology at McMaster University, has been incredibly patient and supportive in guiding the writing of this book.

Barbara Wendland personally would like to thank:

- Janet Chappell, Director of the School of Nutrition at Ryerson University, for the incredible support you provided on this project.
- Dan Mahoney, as well as my other colleagues at Ryerson and my students: you have guided me in more ways than you realize.
- Donna, Carol, and all of my colleagues and friends in the Food and Nutrition Department and beyond at Baycrest — such a caring and humane environment.
- Barry, for your guidance, understanding, and support toward this venture.
- Donna, Minnie, Elizabeth and Sally: you have always been there to guide me.
- My parents for encouraging my sense of curiosity and desire to learn — assets that have been important throughout my life.
- Those who live with acid reflux disease on a daily basis: your experiences have helped me a great deal.
- Lisa Marie, for your energy, vision, and steadfast determination in this project. You created such a wonderful collection of recipes for us all to enjoy!

Lisa Marie Ruffolo personally would like to thank:

- My parents, Carmen and Claudette Ruffolo, for your love and support — and for the use of your kitchen!
- My significant other, David Brennan: your constant encouragement, feedback, and unconditional love mean so much to me.
- Don Douloff, for doing some of the initial recipe testing on a freelance basis.
- My coworkers at Transcontinental Media — especially Lisette Speziale, Christopher Bland, Jeanette Forsythe, Adrian Hayes, and Laurie Brooks Smith — for being so patient and accommodating during this busy time.
- My grandmother, Vilma Vertolli, and my future in-laws, Norma and Patrick Brennan, for your support and for sharing some of your wonderful recipes with me.
- Last, but not least, Barb Wendland, for dedicating your time to help make this book possible.

Index

G

gas, intestinal, 70, 71
gastritis, 45
gastroenterologists, 38
gastroesophageal reflux (GER), 10, 11.
 See also gastroesophageal reflux disease
 (GERD)
 causes, 23–24, 30
 in children, 32, 33
 chronic, 22
 complications, 46
 damage caused by, 15
 doctor's care for, 20, 36–46, 50
 in the elderly, 34
 endoscopy-negative, 36
 obesity and, 28, 35
 in pregnancy, 29–32
 process of, 14–18
 symptoms, 18
 treatments, 19–21, 31–32, 33, 48–54
gastroesophageal reflux disease (GERD),
 11
 diagnosis, 18, 38–45
 erosive, 42, 46
 food reactions in, 85–86
 non-erosive, 46
 prognosis, 45–46
 and quality of life, 36–37, 46
gastroscopy, 38–41
Gaviscon products, 49
grains, 109

H

H. pylori, 45
H2-blockers, 22, 49–50
Health Canada
 Canada's Food Guide to Healthy Eating,
 69, 76, 78–79
 Physical Activity Guide, 62, 63
heart disease, 41
heartburn, 11–12. *See also* gastroesophageal
 reflux (GER)
 body position and, 25, 26
 causes, 23–28
 risk factors, 29–35
Helicobacter pylori, 45
herbal remedies, 51–53
hiatus hernia, 25–26
histamine-2 receptor antagonists (H2-RAs).
 See H-2 blockers
HIV/AIDS, 43

I

ileal brake, 74
immune system, 43
infants, 32, 33

L

lansoprazole (Prevacid), 50
lifestyle changes, 20–21, 31, 57–66
lipids, 74
Losec (omeprazole), 50
lower esphageal sphincter (LES), 12–13, 15,
 24–25

M

Maalox, 48
macronutrients, 68, 69–75, 76–77
manometry, esophageal, 44–45
meal planning, 76–81, 92–112. *See also*
 meals; menus
 for minimal pain, 103–8
 for pain coming under control, 98–103
 for severe pain, 93–98
meals, 58. *See also* diet; foods; meal planning
 content, 25
 eating out, 111–12
 food groups in, 76–77
 frequency, 76
 size, 25, 76
meat and alternatives, 110
medications, 48–53
 adverse reactions to, 41–42
 antacid, 31, 48
 anti-anxiety, 51
 antidepressant, 51, 59
 barrier agent, 31, 32, 49
 bisphosphonate, 42
 herbal, 51–53
 over-the-counter, 18, 19–20, 31, 48–49
 prescribed, 20, 49–50
 troublesome, 27
menus
 for minimal pain, 105–8
 for pain coming under control, 100–103
 for severe pain, 95–98
metoclopramide, 51
micronutrients, 68, 75
milk products, 109
minerals, 75
Mylanta, 48
MyPyramid, 69, 76, 80

Recipe Index

A

appetizers, 124–34
apple
  Apple-Carrot-Cilantro Juice, 224
  Apple Crisp, Lazy, 213
  Applesauce, Easy, 214
  Applesauce-Bran Muffins, 214
  Crimson Sunset Juice, 226
  Pork Tenderloin with Dried Fruit, 176
  Red Cabbage with Apples, 204
  Refreshing Fruit Blend, 225
  Stomach-Aid Juice, 224
  Vegetable Blend, 223
  Waldorf Salad, 152
artichokes
  Artichoke and Potato Stew, 200
  Grilled Chicken with Pesto, 186
  Grilled Veggie Pizza, 163
  Stuffed Sole Fillets, 180
Asian Noodle Soup, 150
Asian Vegetable Stir-Fry, 191
asparagus
  Asparagus and Mushroom Frittata, 116
  Asparagus Gratin, 209
  Spanish Vegetable Paella, 196

B

bacon
  French-Cut Green Beans with Turkey
    Bacon, 207
  Mexican-Style Black Bean Soup, 148
  Truly Canadian Split Pea Soup, 149
Baked Butternut Squash, 198
Baked Chicken Fingers, 169
Baked Haddock, 177
Baked Macaroni and Cheese, 188
Baked Mushroom Caps, 131
Baked Spinach and Rice Casserole, 193
beans, dried
  Fennel Soup, 144
  Mexican-Style Black Bean Soup, 148
  Minestrone, Nonna Vertolli's, 141
  A Taste of Italy Soup, 139
beans, green
  Chicken with Rice, 192
  Creamy Potato Soup (variation), 143
  French-Cut Green Beans with Turkey
    Bacon, 207

Hearty Veal Stew, 175
  Pasta with Peas (variation), 184
  Potato and Green Bean Salad, 155
  Spanish Vegetable Paella, 196
beets
  Crimson Sunset Juice, 226
  Russian-Style Borscht, 147
  Vegetable Blend, 223
bell peppers. See peppers (bell)
Berry Cherry Smoothie, 220
Beta Blend, 208
Beta Power Soup, 138
beverages, 220–26
blueberry
  Berry Cherry Smoothie, 220
  Fruity Splash, 222
  Jam Squares, 218
  Summer Scorcher Smoothie, 221
bread (as ingredient). See also pitas;
    tortillas
  Bread Stuffing, 210
  Five-Minute Meat-on-a-Stick Appetizers,
    127
  French Toast, 121
  Grilled Cheese Sandwich, 160
  Pesto Crostini, 134
  Shrimp Canapés, 128
  Sicilian Spinach Bread, 133
  Tempeh Salad Sandwich, 158
Breaded Veal Cutlets, 174
Breakfast Burritos, 119
Breakfast Potato Patties, 120
Breakfast Quiche, 118
broccoli
  Chinese Broccoli, 206
  Spanish Vegetable Paella, 196
brunch dishes, 116–21

C

cabbage
  Asian Vegetable Stir-Fry, 191
  Chinese Cabbage Rolls, 199
  Creamy Coleslaw, 152
  Crimson Sunset Juice, 226
  Green Cabbage and Potato Blend, 202
  Red Cabbage with Apples, 204
  Russian-Style Borscht, 147
Caribbean Fiesta Dip, 125

Library and Archives Canada Cataloguing in Publication

Wendland, Barbara, 1948–
   Chronic heartburn: managing acid reflux and GERD through understanding, diet and lifestyle / Barbara Wendland, Lisa Marie Ruffolo.

Includes index.
ISBN-13: 978-0-7788-0134-4
ISBN-10: 0-7788-0134-9

1. Heartburn—Popular works. 2. Gastroesophageal reflux—Popular works.
I. Ruffolo, Lisa Marie II. Title.

RC815.7.W45 2005   616.3'2   C2005-906126-X

More Great Books from Robert Rose

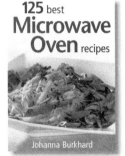

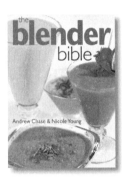

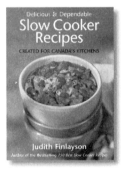

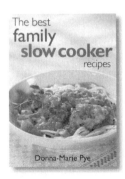

Appliance Cooking

- 125 Best Microwave Oven Recipes
  by Johanna Burkhard
- The Blender Bible
  by Andrew Chase and Nicole Young
- The Mixer Bible
  by Meredith Deeds and Carla Snyder
- The 150 Best Slow Cooker Recipes
  by Judith Finlayson
- Delicious & Dependable Slow Cooker Recipes
  by Judith Finlayson
- 125 Best Vegetarian Slow Cooker Recipes
  by Judith Finlayson
- 125 Best Rotisserie Oven Recipes
  by Judith Finlayson
- 125 Best Food Processor Recipes
  by George Geary
- The Best Family Slow Cooker Recipes
  by Donna-Marie Pye
- The Best Convection Oven Cookbook
  by Linda Stephen
- 125 Best Toaster Oven Recipes
  by Linda Stephen
- 250 Best American Bread Machine Baking Recipes
  by Donna Washburn and Heather Butt
- 250 Best Canadian Bread Machine Baking Recipes
  by Donna Washburn and Heather Butt

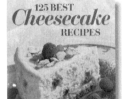

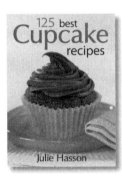

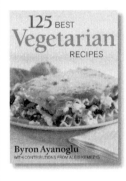

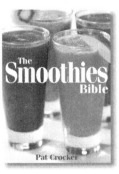

Baking

- 250 Best Cakes & Pies
  by Esther Brody
- 500 Best Cookies, Bars & Squares
  by Esther Brody
- 500 Best Muffin Recipes
  by Esther Brody
- 125 Best Cheesecake Recipes
  by George Geary
- 125 Best Chocolate Recipes
  by Julie Hasson
- 125 Best Chocolate Chip Recipes
  by Julie Hasson
- 125 Best Cupcake Recipes
  by Julie Hasson
- Complete Cake Mix Magic
  by Jill Snider

Healthy Cooking

- 125 Best Vegetarian Recipes
  by Byron Ayanoglu with contributions from Algis Kemezys
- America's Best Cookbook for Kids with Diabetes
  by Colleen Bartley
- Canada's Best Cookbook for Kids with Diabetes
  by Colleen Bartley
- The Juicing Bible
  by Pat Crocker and Susan Eagles
- The Smoothies Bible
  by Pat Crocker